P9-DNY-862

Praise for THE RABBIT EFFECT

"A beautifully written, inspiring book! *The Rabbit Effect* is truly eye-opening and a joy to read. It illuminates vital public health research showing kindness in our day-to-day lives can make the world a healthier, happier place. I recommend this book highly for anyone who wants to live more healthfully."

—**Christy Turlington Burns**, humanitarian and founder of Every Mother Counts

"A wonderful demonstration of how our physical health is affected by the kindness we receive—and the kindness we give. Beautifully written and based on really hard science."

—**Professor Lord Richard Layard**, director of the Well-being Program, Center for Economic Performance at the London School of Economics and Political Science; coauthor of *The World Happiness Report*; and cofounder of Action for Happiness

"[V]ery persuasive. This book provides welcome relief from the over-used and endlessly repeated prescription of diet, sleep, exercise, etc. In a voice that is warm, open, inquisitive, and optimistic, Dr. Harding weaves together compelling clinical vignettes with fascinating medical evidence. This comprehensive, holistic view of health is critical, much needed, and absolutely convincing."

—**Arthur J. Barsky, MD**, professor of psychiatry at Harvard Medical School

"*The Rabbit Effect* is a blockbuster book that will help all of us have a new view of how we create health. It succeeds at putting relationships where they belong: at the center of life, health, and medicine. Dr. Harding shows us that, by being compassionate, giving, and kind human beings, we can win the great rewards of vitality and longevity for ourselves and the whole world. Read this book! It will change your life."

—**Mindy Thompson Fullilove, MD, LFAPA, HonAIA**, author of *Urban Alchemy: Restoring Joy in America's Sorted-Out Cities*

"In this brilliant and delightfully practical book, Dr. Kelli Harding unveils the hidden factors that determine our health and well-being. In a series of fascinating case studies, *The Rabbit Effect* shows how our social environment, from our families to our neighborhoods and workplaces, shapes how we live and whether we heal. Its radical argument is that the most promising remedies for our biomedical problems will come from the social world, not the doctor's office or pharmaceutical lab. *Whether we rebuild it is up to us.*"

—**Eric Klinenberg**, professor of sociology and director of the Institute for Public Knowledge at New York University, and author of *Palaces for the People* and the #1 *New York Times* bestseller *Modern Romance*

"An inspiring, evidence-based, and beautifully written exploration of the profound impact that love, connection, and kindness have on our health. Harding's book should be required reading for all health practitioners and anyone with an interest in living a longer, healthier, and happier life. This is a timely call for a radical rethink in our approach to health care. Compassion and kindness are not fluffy 'nice-to-haves,' they are the vital foundations for our collective well-being and a thriving society."

—**Mark Williamson, PhD**, director of Action for Happiness

"This book is fascinating because of Dr. Kelli Harding's unique ability to combine stories with a deep understanding of the scientific foundation of the stories. This is an extremely compelling book, which will entertain, educate, and impact the readers.

—**Moshe Szyf, PhD**, GlaxoSmithKline and James McGill Professor, Department of Pharmacology & Therapeutics at McGill University Medical School

"It's utterly wonderful. Dr. Harding has reviewed the science on why community matters to individuals' physical and mental health in a truly masterful manner, which will reach both scientific and lay audiences. I learned a great deal."

—**Laurence Guttmacher, MD**, professor of clinical psychiatry, clinical medical humanities, and bioethics at the University of Rochester, School of Medicine & Dentistry

"Dr. Harding knows what our mental health needs. More kindness! This book has a powerful message for us all—backed by ample research—and woven together with the warmth of an expert clinician."

—**Drew Ramsey, MD**, assistant clinical professor of psychiatry at Columbia University and author of *Eat Complete*

"When we first conducted the rabbit studies over forty years ago, we never imagined the critical role that relationships play in health. I'm excited that those studies helped motivate this splendid book. Dr. Harding's evidence-based exploration provides readers with a new way to think about human disease, one rooted in the importance of kindness and relationships. As stated in the Ecclesiastes proverb quoted in the book, a 'faithful friend is the medicine of life.' "

—**Robert M. Nerem, PhD**, professor emeritus, Parker H. Petit Institute for Bioengineering and Bioscience at Georgia Institute of Technology

"Blest are those patients cared for tenderly and wisely by Dr. Kelli Harding. Blest, too, are those who read her book and absorb it into their physical and spiritual lives."

—**Colman McCarthy**, journalist and peace teacher

THE RABBIT EFFECT

THE RABBIT EFFECT

Live Longer, Happier, and

Healthier with the Groundbreaking

Science of Kindness

Kelli Harding, MD, MPH

ATRIA BOOKS

NEW YORK   LONDON   TORONTO   SYDNEY   NEW DELHI

An Imprint of Simon & Schuster, Inc.
1230 Avenue of the Americas
New York, NY 10020

First Atria Books hardcover edition August 2019

ATRIA BOOKS and colophon are trademarks of Simon & Schuster, Inc.

For information about special discounts for bulk purchases, please contact Simon & Schuster Special Sales at 1-866-506-1949 or business@simonandschuster.com.

The Simon & Schuster Speakers Bureau can bring authors to your live event. For more information or to book an event, contact the Simon & Schuster Speakers Bureau at 1-866-248-3049 or visit our website at www.simonspeakers.com.

Interior design by Kyoko Watanabe

Manufactured in the United States of America

10 9 8 7 6 5 4 3 2 1

Library of Congress Cataloging-in-Publication Data

Names: Harding, Kelli, author.
Title: The rabbit effect : live longer, happier, and healthier with the groundbreaking science of kindness / Kelli Harding.
Description: New York : Atria Books, 2019. | Includes bibliographical references.
Identifiers: LCCN 2018059576 (print) | LCCN 2018060169 (ebook) | ISBN 9781501184284 (eBook) | ISBN 9781501184260 (hardback)
Subjects: | MESH: Quality of Life—psychology | Health | Emotional Intelligence | Social Support | Happiness | Empathy
Classification: LCC RA776 (ebook) | LCC RA776 (print) | NLM WA 30 | DDC 613—dc23
LC record available at https://lccn.loc.gov/3018059576

ISBN: 978-1-5011-8426-0
ISBN: 978-1-5011-8428-4 (ebook)

With gratitude for the circles of love and support that surround me:

My parents, for instilling unconditional love. My dad, Bruce, for always cheering me on with unflappable optimism, and my mom, Jacqueline Kerr, for imparting that love knows no boundaries.

My sweet snuggle bunnies, Max, Ryan, and Zay, for teaching me love is limitless. Each of you is a miracle of light and love. Watching you grow is my biggest joy.

Padraic, the dashing stranger from the plane and love of my life, for helping me believe in magic. My life forever changed for the better the day I found you.

My wonderful family and friends who feel like family. You give me endless strength and are close to my heart even when we are far.

My clinician and public health colleagues, for your idealism and unwavering quest to heal human suffering.

My teachers, students, and mentors, for sparking a fire of curiosity and the courage to fan the flames.

My adopted hometown of New York City, for inspiring big wild dreams and making them look doable.

My fellow humans who strive for equity, inclusivity, and peace.

And you, dear reader, for fearlessly creating positive ripples. Your compassion is my inspiration.

We've learned to fly the air like birds.
We've learned to swim the seas like fish.
And yet, we haven't learned to walk
the Earth as brothers and sisters.

—DR. MARTIN LUTHER KING JR.

Contents

THE RABBIT EFFECT

What Are We Missing
in Medicine?

The path to helping people as a doctor seemed straightforward when I arrived at medical school at the University of Rochester. On the first day of my first year, I sat anonymously in the auditorium with ninety-nine other classmates. Clad in spotless white coats, we prepared to cloister ourselves inside the walls of the Strong Memorial Hospital complex. Everything we needed to know about the inner workings of the human body lay within—or so I thought.

For the next four years, my classmates and I followed the well-worn route to the knowledge of medicine: peering through microscopes, cramming for exams in silent library cubicles, and racing through a maze of fluorescent-lit corridors to see patients. During this time, I caught glimpses of daylight reflected off white linoleum. I rarely felt the sun on my skin, the wet grass of spring, or even the bustling city beyond the brick fortress of the hospital complex. Through these intense and completely immersive years, which extended through residency and fellowship, the world outside the hospital seemed irrelevant to my work as a physician. If it weren't for the white rabbits, I might never have walked out the sliding doors of the medical center in search of a new perspective on health.

Introduction

As a medical student on the hospital wards, I noticed odd patterns with patients, observations unmentioned in my medical books. Two patients with the same diagnosis would have two very different courses of illness; one would become gravely ill, while the other carried on an almost normal life. Others I saw had medically unexplained symptoms; I'd search and search, but there was nothing in my texts that supplied a reason for their reported ills. Initially, I felt a vague sense of discomfort with these inconsistencies. I didn't have the narrative or framework to understand them, so I tried to ignore the puzzles they posed. But the nagging feeling that I was missing something in my diagnoses refused to go away. I had accounted for all the usual biomedical explanations. What were the hidden factors in these individuals' health that I wasn't seeing? I was determined to investigate further.

My first suspect was mental health. I wondered if the mysterious interaction of the mind and body could explain why some patients fared better than others. Since no residency-training program addresses the interaction between mental and physical health directly, I self-designed my course of study. First I immersed myself in internal (adult) medicine training at Mount Sinai Hospital in New York City, followed by psychiatry residency training at Columbia University's Irving Medical Center. I remained at Columbia for a National Institute of Mental Health (NIMH) biological psychiatry research fellowship and focused on medically unexplained symptoms. I also became boarded in psychosomatic medicine (consultation-liaison psychiatry). I was a woman on a mission.

Trying to tease apart medical and psychiatric diagnoses is my area of specialty. Clinically, I made the emergency room my home, seeing patients with both acute medical and behavioral concerns. While this means I've seen more than my share of people found naked on New York City streets, it also has provided a front-row seat to both the power and the limits of traditional biomedical knowledge. Despite the fact that I'd trained in a specialty that gave me more insight into people's minds, I still felt I was missing something. Connections between medical symptoms and mental states seemed clear, but why did some people fare so much worse than others when, medically, that shouldn't have been the case? I wanted to understand the different underlying conditions that influence the course of a disease. And then one day, much like Alice, I followed a white rabbit.

"You might want to look at the rabbit studies," Dr. Arthur Barsky suggested. With his carefully side-parted hair, round tortoiseshell glasses, and fatherly demeanor, Arthur was a combination of Clark Kent and a doctor from a black-and-white 1950s medical drama. A member of the Harvard Medical School faculty, and one of my mentors during my fellowship at Columbia, Arthur revealed his secret identity through his research—he, too, was fascinated by medical mysteries. And he dared to question whether answers to a patient's health problems always lie within the traditional boundaries of medicine.

After my fellowship ended, Arthur and I reconnected at a scientific meeting at a symposium I moderated for Dr. Elizabeth Blackburn, the Nobel Prize–winning biologist who discovered the molecular nature of telomeres, the protective caps on our DNA involved in life span. After the meeting, Arthur and I started a series of conversations that began with telomeres and the aging process. Our conference calls, which stretched over years, became a critical part of my education, beyond what's listed on my CV. We brainstormed about clinical curiosities: patients who defied expectations and did well despite terrible diagnoses; curious coincidences such as the increased odds of dying on one's birthday, or in the six months after a spouse dies, or following a broken heart or a surprise party. We discussed patients who get better with inert medications (the placebo effect) and patients who develop severe side effects from pills with no active ingredients (the nocebo effect). How exactly did the mind affect the body? What else might contribute to physical symptoms?

Between our calls, I'd scour the medical literature for studies on the little-understood topics we discussed, such as the relationship between telomere length, premature aging, and life purpose, and then summarize findings for the next discussion. Arthur and I explored the limits of medical understanding, rooted in science and open to possibility. It was Arthur, through his suggestion of the white rabbits, who helped me escape my limited view of health from inside the hospital's cocoon. By then, we'd both become increasingly obsessed with understanding the mystery: *What are we missing in medicine that's crucial to health?*

In medicine, including psychiatry, when we ask what we are missing, we usually find the answer through a research trial or a new drug. The breakthroughs that result from this kind of biomedical research, especially in recent decades, have had substantial consequences for our health. High-tech modern medicine is indisputably superb at keeping someone alive when crisis strikes. Advances in trauma surgery save countless lives. Biomedical advances also transform death sentences into chronic diseases.

What are we missing in medicine that's crucial to health?

In fall 1995 a physician told a razor-thin thirty-seven-year-old man named Robert to get his affairs in order because he had less than a few months left to live. Over two years later, when I attended a fund-raiser in Washington, DC, I met Robert, looking dapper in a tux. Robert's turnaround from AIDS was miraculous. He had put on weight and even developed a bit of a belly, a side effect of the medicine. He bought season tickets to the Kennedy Center with friends and was back to playing Chopin on the piano. The revolutionary class of medication for HIV called protease inhibitors had arrived on the market just in time to save him, and countless others. Many individuals like Robert have discovered life on the other side of a death sentence thanks to biomedical advances.

Yet, despite our scientific progress, Americans are remarkably unhealthy. In 2016 the United States ranked forty-third in the world for life expectancy. Unless we change course, the US is expected to drop to sixty-fourth place by 2040.[1] In 2015 life expectancy for Americans declined for the first time in two decades, while it rose in other wealthy nations. And then the numbers dropped again in 2016 and 2017. During this period, Nobel Prize–winning economist Angus Deaton and his wife, fellow Princeton University professor Anne Case, reported a spike in mortality for middle-aged white men and women with less than a college education. Their data showed that between 1999 and 2013, half a million people died unexpectedly.[2] That's as if the entire population of St. Louis, Missouri, just disappeared.

It's not just life expectancy. America has consistently poor performance on numerous global health measures. For instance, despite spending more than any other country for hospital-based maternity care the US is ranked forty-sixth in the world for maternal health.[3] It also has the worst rate of maternal deaths in the developed world with a rising maternal mortality rate (from 17 deaths per 100,000 births in 2000 to 26.4 deaths per 100,000 in 2015).[4] Compounding the heartache, American children are less likely to reach the age of five than children in other developed countries like Japan. Starting at birth, Americans fall far below other wealthy nations on many standardized health indicators, such as infant mortality, car crashes, mental illness, teen pregnancies, heart disease, imprisonment, homicides, substance use, obesity, and premature death.[5]

America has one of the worst gaps between the health outcomes of rich and poor people, which serves as a key marker of a nation's well-being. Out of the thirty-two wealthiest countries in the world, the US ranked thirty-second on the wealth-health gap.[6] The US is such an outlier of extreme income and health inequality, we are practically not even on the same graph.[7] The same unfortunately holds true for childhood emotional well-being.[8] Even the rich don't live as well as they could. Our comparatively worse health cuts across lines of privilege and race. Wealthy, educated white Americans can expect to die several years younger than equally well-off individuals around the world.[9]

And despite, or perhaps because of, America's status as a global leader in biomedicine, it is also by far the world's most expensive place to get sick. Maybe you or a family member has put off a test or a follow-up visit to save money like one in five Americans.[10] I know I have, even as a doctor working in a hospital. And when we do get sick, the price is outrageous. When my mom died, the cost for her two-week hospital stay totaled well over $100,000. Even with a medical degree, I could barely decipher the bills. Thankfully, she had great insurance and secondary insurance. Through my grief, I understood that we were lucky to be able to pay the remainder; the exorbitant cost of medical care causes half of US bankruptcies annually. One in five of us—including many families with young children—such as those with preemies who require prolonged stays in intensive care units, struggle to pay medical bills.[11]

In the US, the typical solution to health problems, both on an individual and population level, is to double-down on medical care. Problem is, usually, the vast sums of money we spend goes to care *after* we're already sick. It's like towing your car into the shop *after* the brakes have already failed and you've run into a ditch. The cost becomes a vicious circle. Because of the expense, Americans routinely forgo preventive care and don't seek help until it's a five-alarm emergency. Our cost-induced aversion to preventive care, however, only increases the cost of fixing what's wrong when we do seek help. As Dr. Darrell Kirch, president and CEO of the Association of American Medical Colleges, the organization that represents all the accredited US medical schools and major teaching hospitals, said to me, "Good medical care doesn't guarantee good health. There are other factors at work."[12]

Meanwhile, the majority of the $3.5 trillion health-directed resources in the US—more than 95 percent—are spent on clinical care–related services.[13] This includes doctor's office visits, hospital stays, medications, imaging studies, laboratory testing, and procedures (i.e., biopsies, surgeries, etc.), nursing care facilities, and related administrative costs. What's strange is our government spends absurd amounts of money on these services compared to every other developed country in the world, and still one in ten Americans does not have health coverage.[14] America dedicates nearly twice as much of its economy to health care as the UK (17.9 percent US GDP versus 9 percent UK GDP), yet, unlike the British, we don't provide basic free medical care for all.[15] It's like we've walked into a supermarket where the cashier charges us double for the same apples as everyone else, and ours are rotten.

It's like we've walked into a supermarket where the cashier charges us double for the same apples as everyone else, and ours are rotten.

For me as doctor, there's one more point that's truly shocking. Data shows that clinical care, as we currently provide it, isn't actually making us much healthier. In fact, studies estimate that what happens at the doctor's office and hospital accounts for only 10 to 20 percent of a person's overall health status; it doesn't significantly contribute to overall population health and well-being. Additionally, evidence shows spending more on medical care access and quality only improves preventable deaths by a slim 10 to 15 percent.[16] Despite our massive investment in health care, numerous well-done studies paint the same picture over and over: the contribution of medical measures to the decline in mortality is questionable.[17]

> **Our nation spends a fortune on health care, yet we remain remarkably unwell.**

These surprising findings are at the heart of this book. Our nation spends a fortune on health care, yet we remain remarkably unwell.

So if biomedical advances and expensive medical care aren't making the difference to our health, what is? What would actually make us healthier?

Which brings us to the rabbits.

New Zealand white male rabbits develop heart disease much like humans if fed a high-fat diet. Today most people know that eating fried food and steaks daily is asking for trouble. But back in 1978, researchers were still trying to establish the relationship between high blood cholesterol and heart health. Dr. Robert Nerem and his team designed a straightforward experiment using what he calls "the standard rabbit model" to show the link.[18] Over several months, he fed a group of rabbits the same high-fat diet. At the end of the study, he measured the animals' cholesterol, heart rates, and blood pressure. As expected, the cholesterol values were all high and virtually identical to one another. The rabbits had similar genes and ate the same diet. Now they all seemed destined for a heart attack or stroke.

As the last step, Dr. Nerem needed to examine the rabbits' tiny blood vessels. Looking through the microscope, he expected all the rabbits to show similar fatty deposits on the inside of their arteries. Instead, Dr. Nerem had a shock. As it turned out, there was a huge variation in the fatty deposits between the animals. One group of rabbits had 60 percent fewer deposits than the other. It made no sense. He recalls wondering, "What in the world could this be?" There was no clear biological explanation for these findings. He was staring down his microscope at a medical mystery.

Dr. Nerem and his team searched for clues. They looked again at the research design. Nothing unusual. But Dr. Nerem knew to keep looking. He said, "Sometimes there are things involved in a protocol that we don't take into account." So the research team looked at themselves.

A Canadian postdoc named Murina Levesque had recently joined the lab. Dr. Nerem remembers, "She was an unusually kind and caring individual." When it became apparent that all the animals with fewer fatty deposits were under Murina's care, the team dug deeper. They noticed that Murina handled the animals differently. When she fed her rabbits, she talked to them, cuddled and petted them. She didn't just pass out rabbit kibble—she gave them love. As Dr. Nerem explains, "She couldn't help it. It's just how she was."

Now a professor emeritus of bioengineering at Georgia Tech, Dr. Nerem says, "We were not social behavioral scientists," but the team decided they could not ignore the findings of the social environment's effect on physiology. The research group repeated the experiment, this time with tightly controlled conditions. They compared the arteries of one group of rabbits cared for by the new postdoc to the arteries of another group of rabbits cared for in the standard way. They found the same effect again and published these findings in the prestigious journal *Science*.[19] Take a rabbit with an unhealthy lifestyle. Talk to it. Hold it. Give it affection. And many adverse effects of diet disappear. The relationship made a difference. *But how?*

Medical training teaches doctors to break the body down into disparate parts: organs, tissues, cells, and molecules. Physicians divide by specialty in this same way. There are doctors for every bit: heart, kidney, gut, bone, brain, and so on. This fragmented view stems from the underlying theoretical premise that disease arises from internal biological processes gone haywire. It is an exciting inner-world journey that has dominated medical thinking for the last century, and it is what I—and countless other medical doctors—spent all those years painstakingly studying.

But then there were the rabbits. These studies indicate something is missing in the traditional biomedical model. It wasn't diet or genetics that made a difference in which rabbits got sick and which stayed healthy; it was kindness.

It turns out the rabbits were just the introduction to a much larger story. I call it the Rabbit Effect.

When it comes to our health, we've been missing some crucial pieces: hidden factors behind what really makes us healthy. Factors like love, friendship, and dignity. The designs of our neighborhoods, schools, and workplaces. There's a social dimension to health we've completely overlooked in our scramble to find the best and most cutting-edge personalized medical care. Even having something that motivates us to get up and out of bed in the morning makes a difference to our physical well-being.

Because, as it turns out, being and staying healthy isn't something that can be addressed through biomedical advances alone. Or by more and more spending on health care. Even the usual self-help directives—"Eat better! Work out! Get more sleep!"—will only get us so far. All these approaches overlook the critical social dimensions to ensuring sound minds and bodies. Ultimately, what affects our health in the most meaningful ways has as much to do with how we treat one another, how we live, and how we think about what it means to be human than with anything that happens in the doctor's office.

This book will empower you to change your health. But not in the usual ways. I won't give you a ten-step fitness plan or a two-week diet. That's not what you need. That's not going to make you healthier in the long run. Instead, I'll take you with me through the halls of the hospital, invite you into the room with my patients to discover why they are sick and what might make them well. Together, we'll investigate clinical puzzles that defy expectations, unearthing the hidden factors that determine who is sick and who is well, who will live and who will thrive. We'll discuss stories from communities renowned for their

This book will empower you to change your health. But not in the usual ways.

longevity, and data from studies that turn conventional thinking on its head.

We'll also explore the surprisingly strong connection between mental and physical health. Together let's examine how that physiological link, in turn, is aggravated by hidden factors awry in our environment. In other words, to better understand why and how we get sick—and how individuals can boost health—we'll look at the brain and body in the context of our day-to-day interactions. We'll then zoom out to an aerial view and look at solutions that boost collective health for all of us. At the end of each chapter there is a tool kit that offers ideas for your own process of self-discovery.

None of this means I'm going to insist you see a therapist. Or try to convince you to take more pills. Instead, we'll learn to pay attention to how symptoms, such as anxiety or depression or fatigue or pain, may reflect a red flag that something going on in your world needs attention. And how once we've addressed our own red flags, we can individually and collectively help others address theirs.

Ultimately, we will come to see how the larger ties that bind us—ties of love, connection, purpose—have ripple effects on our health and the world at large. And throughout the process, we'll consider fundamental questions about how we live. I'll ask you to examine your family, your relationships, your community, your neighborhood, your work, and your passions. I'm going to ask you to forget everything you think you know about health and wellness, and together we'll open our minds to a new paradigm, a new way of thinking about how we live and what it means to thrive.

THE HIDDEN FACTORS

Chapter One

The Hidden Factors of Health

You are my other me. If I do harm to you, I do harm to myself.
If I love and respect you, I love and respect myself.
—LUIS VALDEZ

Let's begin with a story. It's a tale of two patients, Bella and Daisy, which illustrates how the best of health and the worst of health are not always what they seem.

Looking at Bella's medical record, it was clear she was gravely ill. At seventy, she was diagnosed with pancreatic cancer, a particularly aggressive disease that often results in weight loss and jaundice. At the time of her diagnosis, Bella was surprised to learn that she was so sick. Though she traveled a long road through surgery, chemotherapy, and radiation, three years later, at seventy-three, she looked radiant and seemed surprisingly youthful. Bella showed up to her doctor's visits wearing sporty sneakers. She often spent her Saturdays out in the yard tending her marigolds, going to art classes, or taking a stroll with her son, who lived down the street. She was glad when the chemotherapy ended so she could invite her neighbor and the woman's two young daughters over for freshly baked chocolate chip oatmeal cookies, or "cowgirl cookies," as she called them, her specialty. Her main complaint was that one of her medicines made her more susceptible to sunburn.

Unlike Bella, Daisy had a squeaky-clean bill of health on paper. All her bloodwork, imaging, and cardiac tests came back normal. Though she was almost half Bella's age, at forty-three, Daisy looked withered and acted much older. Her face held traces of beauty faded by forces unknown. She moved slowly and sighed when she sat down. At each clinic visit, she said she felt "foggy" and exhausted all the time. She lacked the energy to leave her house or travel to see her favorite cousin, Viola, who had recently moved to Pennsylvania. She had a variety of unaccounted for aches and pains and had missed so many days in her job as a paralegal that she had no more vacation or sick time left. Bella would ask despondently, "I just don't feel right. Do you think we've missed something?"

In Western medicine, sick and well are often viewed in black and white, or as mutually exclusive buckets. In the biomedical model—medicine's dominant twentieth-century view that physical factors alone explain human health—a doctor tells Bella, a woman who feels fine but has a suspicious lab finding, that she is sick and needs medical treatment. Meanwhile, Daisy, who feels sick yet has no concerning findings, is assured all is well, perhaps told that what she is experiencing is only in her head, and sent home. Both patients leave the clinic confused.

During my research fellowship exploring medically unexplained symptoms, I saw patients who were ostensibly well, but felt lousy—or who worried they were ill to the point that they couldn't function in life. Many patients had gone from doctor to doctor or ER to ER looking for an answer. The mismatch between how a person feels and their doctor's findings is perplexing. This was the odd pattern I'd discussed with Arthur Barsky during our phone calls that had led me to the rabbits. How can someone be medically ill and feel well? Or be well and feel ill? Is there a way to think about health that accounts for both situations?

Dr. George Engel, an internist at the University of Rochester School of Medicine, posed a daring answer. On April 8, 1977, *Science* published an article in which Dr. Engel questioned the widely held belief in American medicine that biology alone explains human illness. Dr. Engel saw medicine marching along on a narrowly focused quest for physical markers of disease divorced from the broader context of human life. He warned that the ideology of the entrenched biomedical model was the "crippling flaw" of the field and not enough to explain human health.[1] An incomplete truth adopted as a dangerous dogma.

As a physician, Dr. Engel was puzzled by the gray zone between sick and well. He felt the explanation of the gray zone might come from more closely examining "the patient and his attributes as a person, as a human being." In short, Dr. Engel thought the difference between patients like Bella and Daisy might involve examining their lives with a much wider lens than any instrument you'd find in a doctor's office.

Influenced by Dr. Adolf Meyer at Johns Hopkins University, general systems theory, and fields outside of medicine, Dr. Engel proposed a broader, more inclusive concept of health that took a patient's whole life into account. It unified biomedicine and behavioral health into a complete package. Dr. Engel called his new theory the biopsychosocial model. While the name is a mouthful, the concept is simple. The idea is that a person's health occurs in a social context that can't be ignored.

The biopsychosocial model (see figure 1) systematically organizes the layers of health. Nothing exists in isolation: each layer is both simultaneously a whole and a part. A shift in one part affects change elsewhere. The innermost parts contain the molecules, organelles, cells, tissues, organs, and nervous system that comprise a person. This is where the biomedical model and health-care system stop. Dr. Engel saw that, though the vast majority of medical practice is focused on the inner layers alone, health extends far beyond the body.

Looking at individual biology in isolation provides an incomplete picture that makes the cases of Bella and Daisy perplexing. Why is "sick" Bella doing so great and "well" Daisy doing so poorly? If you expand out through the rings, the cases of Bella and Daisy make more sense. When we take the factors in Dr. Engel's outer rings, the rings beyond the "person level," into account, we start to see the grave differences in Bella's and Daisy's situations and thus their health. It reminds me of the stretchy portraits on the walls of the Haunted Mansion at Disneyland, where initially, you see just a painting of a lovely young woman with a bucolic smile holding a parasol. But then the picture frame stretches out to reveal her standing on a tightrope over the open jaws of a crocodile.

Keeping with the idea that health extends far beyond the body alone,

DR. ENGEL'S BIOPSYCHOSOCIAL MODEL
CONTINUUM OF NATURAL SYSTEMS

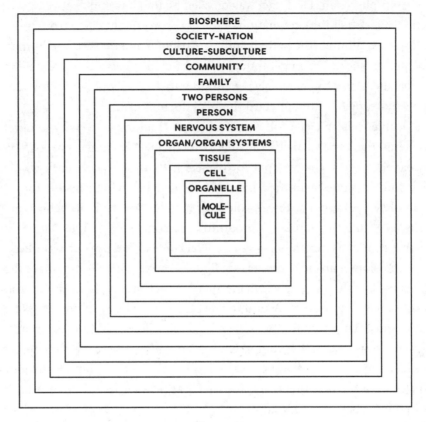

Figure 1

G. L. Engel, "The Clinical Application of the Biopsychosocial Model,"
American Journal of Psychiatry 137, no. 5 (May 1980): 535–44.

Dr. Engel's model stretches outward from the individual to include a two-person relationship, family, community, culture, society-nation, and biosphere. The outer layers contain the psychological and social factors that I, along with most of my physician colleagues, considered irrelevant or intrusive while hiding out in the medical center with my patients. With a complete picture, we start to see how "sick" Bella's well-being connects to her strolls with her son, sense of community, and favorite hobbies. And how "well" Daisy's poor health relates to her isolation, missing her cousin Viola, and a lack of engagement at work.

Dr. Engel, who often wore a red bow tie on his rounds at the University of Rochester School of Medicine, practiced what he preached. Those who knew him said he always noticed not just a patient's physical findings but little details about her life, such as if she had family pictures up in her hospital room or flowers delivered by friends. He was the kind of trusted doctor you'd feel relieved to see and welcome into the room with a sick family member. He'd sit down to talk with the person not just about medical problems, but about her life and priorities. He built a large consultation service to address the holistic needs of hospitalized patients, including psychological and social factors. Though Dr. Engel died at age eighty-five, at the beginning of my medical training in Rochester, his legacy of taking the time to get to know patients as human beings permeates the medical school culture and its graduates.

In fact, Dr. Engel's model was one of the first things I was introduced to in medical school. On that first day of my first year, at the front of the room stood Dr. Edward Hundert, the dean of students and a mentee of Dr. Engel. In his understated, wise way, Dr. Hundert introduced us to the biopsychosocial model. Without much fanfare, he walked us through the realms of the human condition. He explained that the model served as the basis of our medical school curriculum at Rochester and would be invaluable in our care for patients going forward.

I paused—for a moment.

But then my classmates and I got down to the real business of studying what we had come to learn: biomedicine. It seemed every class we took, every book we read, and every patient we saw echoed the same gospel. Diagnose the body. Treat the body. I thought my doctor's bag held my superpower—medications. Chemical structure of Treatment A, predicted binding at Receptor B, and improvement of symptoms for Disease C. By the time I had completed all my exams and started seeing patients on the clinical wards, I'd forgotten all about learning Dr. Engel's model and the broader context of illness. I craved experience and felt curious with excitement to see the diseases I'd only studied in books.

And then I met Randy.

Randy was only forty-seven, but looked a decade older. He had a kid-with-a-hand-in-the-cookie-jar smile with brown crooked teeth, and long curly black hair with a bald spot on top. He'd led a rock-and-roll life as a stage manager for a popular city nightclub. In his twenties, he did heroin intravenously. While he'd managed to kick that habit, he'd taken to smoking a pack and a half of cigarettes a day. "The lesser of two evils," as he described it. He also liked to have two shots of whiskey to "get going" in the evenings.

By his late thirties, Randy's prized concert tour T-shirt collection was too tight to wear. A doctor diagnosed him with type 2 diabetes. He was supposed to inject himself with long-acting insulin but wasn't too strict about it. His girlfriend, Sherri, pointed out that with his late nights, Randy had always had a hard time keeping up with his medications and ate mostly bar food. By the age of forty-two, he noticed a painful cramping in his legs would come and go as he was climbing theater stairs or a ladder setting up for a show. Then the cramping started happening when he was just standing around talking with the crew. At forty-four, he developed an ulcer on his big toe that wouldn't heal. That toe was his first amputation.

By the afternoon I met Randy, he had significantly advanced peripheral vascular disease. Earlier that year he'd had femoral popliteal bypass surgery, or "fem-pop," to try to circumvent a blockage in the major artery of his leg. In a delicate four-hour procedure, the vascular surgery team removed Randy's functioning saphenous vein and carefully restitched it at the femoral artery above and below his left knee. When the procedure goes well, the bypass improves blood flow to the lower leg. The surgery was a success, without a single complication. Randy was expected to do well.

Six months later, Randy had a new infection on his lower left leg. I stopped by his hospital room with my senior resident, Dr. Brian Cooper, whom the team called "Coop," to take a look. As we removed the bandages on the pale cold leg, the stench was unbearable. Randy's wound looked as bad as it smelled. Because of his bad circulation, what had started as a tiny cut from the corner of a metal coffee table had become a festering sore. Randy looked at me as I looked at the leg. I breathed through my mouth and tried to maintain a professional veneer as I concealed my horror. Because of Randy's blocked circulation, the intravenous antibiotics could not reach the wound site to work. Treatment A could not bind at Receptor B. If the antibiotic couldn't reach Randy's leg, there would be no improvement of Disease C. He would die from the infection.

Randy sat in his hospital bed. Sherri sat at his side reading a celebrity magazine. Coop was blunt. "Are you still smoking?"

Randy chuckled. "Is Mick Jagger still with the Stones?"

Coop did not crack a smile. Randy's fingers were yellow with tobacco stains. "You understand, smoking prevents the tissues from properly healing after a surgery." Nicotine both weakens the body's fighter immune cells and is a vasoconstrictor, preventing the cells from getting to the site of trauma. It's like drugging soldiers and then putting them in a tank on a blocked road. Randy explained that even if he didn't smoke, everyone else at his job did. Coop continued, "We'll do several tests this afternoon to check the blood flow to your foot and then talk about our options. I have to be frank. From the look of that leg, I'm not optimistic."

Randy had other questions on his mind. "Hey, Doc, is there anything we can do about this?" and he pointed to his pelvic area. He leaned over to us and in a loud whisper said, "The diabetes is really killin' my love life." Sherri sheepishly nodded. Coop put a hand on his shoulder and said, "One thing at a time, sir." The reality was, that was not our area.

After we exited the room, Coop shook his head. He summed up the situation: "If a fem-pop flops, then it's a chop-chop." He made a chopping motion with his arm on his own thigh. "And there, it don't stop," moving up his leg. By evening, the tests confirmed the obvious. The femoral bypass had failed. We shared the news with Randy. It wasn't safe for him to leave the hospital with his left leg intact. Because of the extent of the infection, we'd put him on the schedule for an above-the-knee amputation first thing the next morning. Randy looked at his hands as he took in the news and nodded. We all sat quietly. Sherri cried. Eventually he asked, "Can someone wheel me outside for a smoke?"

I've asked myself many times how Randy might have avoided losing that leg and what else we could have done to prevent further catastrophe. Most clinicians know in their gut that treating a person's leg or body with medical or surgical care alone isn't enough to ensure health. Dr. Engel had encouraged us to look at our patients' lives. But lives are messy, and asking something off-script feels like cracking open the lid on Pandora's box in a fifteen-minute visit. Our current system says stick to the leg, so that's what we do. And yet when I looked at Randy—at his bad diet, his smoking, his inability to take the medicines prescribed, why a small injury led to a festering sore—it was hard not to feel like the answer lay in his life. And not just his life, but in a more systematic examination of the currents that had shaped his health upstream.

To better understand those upstream forces, I crossed the street from the medical center and enrolled in classes at Columbia University's Mailman School of Public Health. Sitting in seminars with people from all different backgrounds, not just physicians, I felt I'd entered a parallel universe where everyone was talking about health but in a radically different way. Medicine and public health are strangely two separate worlds that look at health from two very different perspectives. Like Alice, I'd passed through the looking glass. On the clinical side, Dr. Engel's model said a patient's life matters to her health, and on the public health side, I saw that the field had a far more in-depth understanding of the specific conditions that shape our lives, and thus a person's behavior and biology. But the two halves needed unification with a common language.

From my new perspective, I saw clearly that the field of public health illuminated what Dr. Engel started. Since Dr. Engel's landmark paper, more than forty years of medical, public health, and scientific research on the social dimensions of disease show that he was right: the vast majority, 80 to 90 percent, of people's health depends on factors outside clinical care.[2] While genes do play a role (more on that later) the biggest contributor to health outcomes by far are powerful social, political, and environmental conditions. It turns out that where a person is born, works, lives, plays, and grows older—what the field of public health calls the *social determinants of health*—shape a person's behavior and biology in profound ways. The social determinants, or hidden factors, of health are the "risks of risks," or the conditions under which

> Where a person is born, works, lives, plays, and grows older shape a person's behavior and biology in profound ways.

disease strengthens or withers.[3] It is not the language that Dr. Engel used, but it defines what he described.

By marrying Dr. Engel's elegant biopsychosocial model with the commonsense language of the social determinants, I moved closer to solving the puzzle of not just Randy, but Bella and Daisy and so many others. The key to understanding why they—and we—aren't healthier lay in a new framework, a framework I call the "hidden factors." It unifies not only the fields of medicine and mental health, but makes a substantial leap to include the vast world of public health too. And it also involves you. The hidden factors model brings us back to that first day of medical school and Dr. Hundert's sage, yet unheeded, advice from orientation that considering the broader human condition is critical for health.

In the rings of the hidden factors (see figure 2), at the center is the individual: you. Radiating outward from you is the social and environmental matrix in which you participate every moment of every day. This framework incorporates everything in our lives: family, friends, coworkers, money, vacations, schools, hobbies, homes, sidewalks, streetlights, grocery stores, coffee shops, hairdressers, parks, playgrounds, community centers, places of worship, transportation, times of reflection, and how we navigate one another. It's all the activities of our daily lives.

In the chapters that follow, we'll explore the rings of the hidden factors model together. The first ring, closest to oneself, looks at our one-on-one relationships, or our most intimate bonds. Then we'll look at the vital role of broader social ties in our health and communities. Where and how we work is also critical to our health and well-being, and it dovetails with our education, or learning, and our greater sense of life purpose. Next, we'll travel to our neighborhood, and examine where we live and play. How we treat each other, or living by the "Golden Rule," is essential to creating a culture where we can all thrive with fairness. As we get to the outer edges, we take a look at broader factors, like our environmental influences and specifically childhood exposures that impact the mind and body. And last, we'll delve into how emotional well-being, trust, and conflict resolution skills help all of us live in healthier and more peaceful societies. It's an eye-opening journey with pressing implications for our daily choices.

THE SOCIAL DIMENSIONS OF HEALTH: THE HIDDEN FACTORS

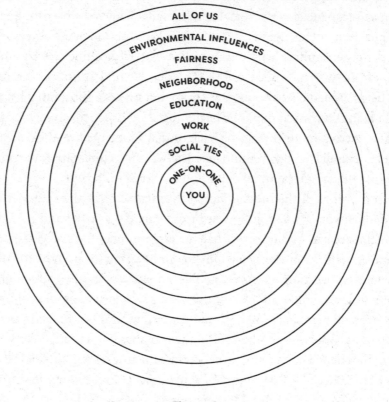

ALL OF US

ENVIRONMENTAL INFLUENCES

FAIRNESS

NEIGHBORHOOD

EDUCATION

WORK

SOCIAL TIES

ONE-ON-ONE

YOU

Figure 2

All these hidden factors were present in Randy's life. In fact, they help explain how Randy got as sick as he did, and why a tiny cut turned into a festering sore. What if his doctors had been trained to treat these factors when Randy first sought care? What if our medical systems considered addressing hidden factors early as part of routine visits and got patients the support they needed? Prevention in medicine reminds me of time travel movies, like *Back to the Future*, where tiny changes to early events lead to shifts in destiny. As it was, Randy was lucky to only lose the leg. In a different version where hidden factors were addressed early, maybe Randy wasn't stuck in a hospital bed awaiting surgery.

Here are some of the ways Randy's story could have gone differently. Starting with his closest relationships, he was lucky. He had a huge social support in Sherri. But Sherri needed support, too, and she could have helped us help Randy. A high priority should have been to help Randy stop smoking, or at least cut back. After all, each additional cigarette reduces a person's life by 11 minutes.[4] But beyond an appointment at a smoking cessation clinic, it also would have helped to know that Randy's passion was electric guitar repair. Understanding that was important to him and connecting him to classes may have ultimately provided a better work environment and a healthier sleep schedule. Work and learning are only two hidden factors we'll discuss that could have changed the course of Randy's health.

And here's the thing: Randy isn't the exception. He's the rule. Take Carl. Carl may on the surface need a straightforward "hernia repair." But he's also an older man living alone, with uncontrolled hypertension, a flight of stairs he can't navigate, and unreliable transportation to his doctors' appointments. Or Sandra has a "bowel obstruction." But she's also a single mother of three, living in a one-bedroom apartment, who prioritizes her kids' needs over her own pricey medications. Meanwhile, Sean has a bulging "cervical herniated disc," but also feels trapped in a stressful public relations job with a boss who's a major pain in the neck. Gloria needs a "cholecystectomy" (her gallbladder removed), but she also needs to get out of her abusive marriage.

Illuminating the hidden factors helps us see where to focus our efforts to improve our health. They explain why the same course of treatment or medications for a disease can lead to very different outcomes. Clinically, it's common to see two patients with the same condition, such as recovering after a heart attack, have two very different courses based on seemingly irrelevant factors, such as their family relationships or their education level. In my practice, the sickest people I see often share similar backgrounds: loneliness, abuse, poverty, or discrimination. For them, the medical model isn't enough. It's like fixing up an airplane engine and ignoring that the pilot is on his third drink at the bar and a massive storm is overhead.

The narrow focus of our current medical model may enable doctors to fix specific problems; but while fixing something that's broken is immensely satisfying, it's not a lasting solution if we don't take the whole person and the context of their life into account. To properly care for patients, we also need to care about the lives of the people getting the care. A competent surgeon can perform a successful femoral bypass on Randy's leg, but it will ultimately fail unless the necessary everyday supports are in place. We may fix the problem, but we fail the patient. The flip side is that if we can address the different rings of the hidden factors early, tackle the risks of risks, illness might never progress to the extremes we see daily in the ER. This message needs to be heard far beyond the walls of the hospital, as we lose lives full of promise every day to preventable causes. It seems the essentials of health rest not in medical textbooks, but in our everyday connections to each other.

We may fix the problem, but we fail the patient.

What we are missing in medicine is that health extends far beyond the body alone and includes our social world. During the course of our lifetimes, we'll all inevitably find ourselves in the mystery zone between health and illness like Bella and Daisy. How can we enjoy good health no matter what may come? To explore this question, let's travel through the concentric rings of the hidden factors together. How we treat each other as human beings matters deeply for our health, so we'll start with our closest relationships.

It seems the essentials of health rest not in medical textbooks, but in our everyday connections to each other.

Chapter Two

One-on-One:
Your Intimate Relationships

*If you want to change the world, go
home and love your family.*
—MOTHER TERESA

Twins often arrive early. While most single births remain in the womb for about forty weeks, the average twin pregnancy is only thirty-five weeks. When Kate Ogg went into labor at twenty-seven weeks, she knew her twins were in grave danger. The girl, named Emily, survived birth. The boy, named Jamie, did not. The doctors tried everything to get him to breathe, but after twenty minutes, they pronounced the baby dead. The doctors told the family that nothing more could be done to save him. Before the staff took him out of the room, Kate asked permission to hold her son.

Kate unwrapped the baby's blanket and placed Jamie, with his paper-thin skin, on her chest. Her husband, David, lay in the hospital bed with them. David took off his shirt for extra warmth next to the baby. They were both in tears. As they sat huddled together, skin-to-skin, Kate talked to her son. "We explained his name and that he had a twin that he had to look out for and how hard we tried to have him," Kate said in an interview with the *Telegraph*.[1] And then it happened.

Jamie began moving in short bursts. The midwife explained this was a reflex of the dying. Then his eyes suddenly opened, possibly another reflex. Kate thought Jamie looked around. The staff reminded the family that they needed to let him go. As Kate and David continued to hold and talk to him, Jamie seemed to be breathing. Then, he reached out a hand and grasped David's finger. They excitedly called out for the doctor, who didn't return.

Over the next hour, Jamie continued to grow stronger. As Kate recounted on a *Today* show interview, her husband eventually said, "Go tell [the doctor] we've come to terms with the baby's death, can he just come and explain it?" She added, "That made him come back."[2] Five years later, news reports show Jamie as a happy child with sandy blond hair and a broad smile. He likes to run on the beach near his family's home in Sydney, Australia, play games, make silly faces, and bake cookies with his sister.[3]

What happened that day with Jamie was an extraordinary situation, and we may never know exactly what occurred. But we do know a baby pronounced dead showed glimmers of life as he lay snuggled against his mother's and father's skin. His parents' loving touch somehow changed everything. Or so it seemed. The doctors focused only on Jamie's tiny body. But larger hidden factors, including parental love, were at play.

How could a mother's love change a child's destiny? As a young man studying philosophy in college, Dr. Moshe Szyf wondered about "very, very old questions." Is behavior shaped by experience (such as love) or biology (such as genetics)? As time passed, Dr. Szyf studied genetics at Harvard and eventually became a professor of pharmacology and therapeutics at McGill University, working on cancer research. He never imagined how, years later, his early interest in philosophy would reemerge in a bar in Madrid. That Spanish night in 1992, drinking a couple of pints after a conference with a university colleague, Dr. Michael Meaney, the conversation turned to rats.

Working in his lab, Dr. Meaney had noticed some rats made more loving mothers than others. The more nurturing rat moms lick their babies a lot during the first week postpartum, while the more emotionally distant spend little time grooming their offspring. Dr. Meaney observed that "high lickers" raise more relaxed pups that are docile, whereas "low lickers" produce more anxious pups that are hard to handle and may even bite. Anyone in the lab could easily pick out the rat mother's parenting style based on the pup's behavior. Additionally, the mother's style seemed to dictate the pup's behavior for life. Dr. Szyf was intrigued. He told me, "As a scientist, I'm looking for things that seem strange and different."[4] Now he wondered about one of the oldest questions on earth: How does nurture shape our nature? If genetics are fixed, why was love changing personality?

Dr. Szyf, Dr. Meaney, and their colleagues designed an ingenious experiment to find out if a mother's nurturing behavior made the difference to the rat baby even if the baby and the mom had different genetic makeups. Since rats are happy to foster other mothers' babies, the researchers swapped the pups. Then the team tediously counted rat licks. What they found was as strong an argument for nurture over nature as

If genetics are fixed, why was love changing personality?

any: if the daughter of a low-licker anxious rat was raised by a high-licker relaxed mom, she became a relaxed rat. Eventually, she would go on to be a high-licker mom, too, raising relaxed pups. The opposite held true as well.[5]

Was it possible that with each additional lick, the mother was reshaping the baby's genetic script? This idea rocked Dr. Szyf's understanding of genetics. The answer would reveal the amazing flexibility of life, and he grew determined to figure out how that worked.

Strangely enough, a Nazi-induced famine in the Netherlands during World War II may hold some of the answers. In October 1944, only months after the Gestapo discovered Anne Frank and sent her to Auschwitz, Nazi forces abruptly cut off food supplies to over four million Dutch citizens, including women and children, living in the western Netherlands. There was not enough bread or milk to feed everyone, and over twenty thousand people died of starvation. Those who survived the "hunger winter" did so mostly thanks to airdropped food programs, such as Operation Chowhound and Operation Manna, by neighboring Allied countries. But 400 to 800 calories a day is insufficient nutrition, especially for expectant mothers.

After the Nazi forces in Norway surrendered on May 5, 1945, food supplies rapidly returned to normal levels. But the catastrophic famine left a hidden mark. Researchers who wished to understand the impact of a mother's diet during pregnancy on her baby's health discovered it. In the Netherlands, citizens' collective health is tracked over time in a database known as a public health registry. A registry provides valuable data on the health of a population. (In the US, with our fragmented medical system and millions of medical records that don't communicate with one another, we do not have anything as extensive.) Thanks to the country-wide registry, the birth records of babies conceived or in utero during the famine provided valuable clues to health investigators.

What the investigators found may not sound so dramatic in and of itself: mothers most affected by the famine had smaller-than-average babies. But what's surprising is that the babies' small size was only the beginning. Researchers tracked these low-weight babies into adulthood. As they grew older, the Dutch Famine cohort went on to develop more health problems, such as increased risk of heart disease, obesity, diabetes, and mental illness.[6] They died years younger than those born before or after the famine.[7] Some studies showed even the following generation—the famine babies' babies—had low weights, suggesting the effects of a grandmother's starvation were passed down through multiple generations. The environment was having a long-term impact. Not getting enough food one winter echoed at least two generations down the line. A subsequent study published in Cell replicated these findings in rats and found eating habits in pregnancy did pass down three generations.[8]

But how exactly does it work? Famine doesn't change a fixed DNA sequence. How could an environmental trauma rewrite the genetic script and pass it on?

Before the rat licking studies, Dr. Szyf serendipitously studied DNA methylation, a process he'd seen in tumor cells. Like a period added to a sentence, methylation attaches a methyl group (CH_3) to the DNA strand and signals pauses during transcription, or the process of gene expression. DNA methylation is known as an *epigenetic* process, meaning it's in addition to the genes.[9] The methyl group is separate from the DNA strand itself.

Methylation alters the cell's narrative without changing the genetic code. Instead, it twists and turns the DNA story into a new, sometimes better or sometimes worse plot line. With cancer cells, it can transform a lighthearted romantic comedy into a tearjerker. Whereas, with positive lifestyle changes, even if someone has a sinister plot line written into his DNA, alterations in methylation can slow down the progression of the story for the better. This means a person may live healthier longer before symptoms of a disease, such as with neurodegenerative illnesses (including Alzheimer's, Parkinson's, and Huntington's diseases), begin to emerge.[10] It turns out our DNA is far more flexible than we thought.

Dr. Szyf had never imagined that the social environment could influence methylation. Then, in a fortuitous twist, Dr. Szyf and his team's laboratory analysis saw DNA methylation and de-methylation occur with the rat mother's neglect or love of her child. Exposure to love or neglect embedded in the baby's body on a microscopic level, and it seemed to pass on. In other words, as Dr. Szyf explained with delight, he had found, "Experience embedded in the genome!"

Through the flexible epigenetic process, environmental exposures flip genes on and off to adapt to life's unfolding drama. For example, when a baby grows in his mother's womb, stress hormones, such as cortisol, cross the placenta. The stress doesn't change the fixed DNA code itself, but through methylation passes a vital message to the developing life on how to arrange DNA for immediate survival: "It's a rough world out there, kid, get ready!" It seems epigenetics is like fashion. A bikini or a winter coat transforms the person, and if it's summer in Miami or winter in Montreal, it could mean life or death.

The Dutch Famine cohort and Dr. Szyf's rat pups aren't the only babies studied whose genes were affected by their experiences. An unexpected Canadian snowstorm offers even more insight into how exactly the epigenetic process works.

For residents of Quebec and Eastern Ontario with a heavy winter coat, snow is no big deal. Life stays in motion: schools are open, work is business as usual, and traffic hums along. During January 1998, however, five small winter storms ganged up to create one humongous disaster. In the Great Canadian Ice Storm of 1998, trees toppled onto cars and houses, live power lines snapped, and transmission towers collapsed. Thirty-five people died. Bridges and tunnels closed, leaving millions of people stranded without electricity for up to six weeks.[11] Montreal became paralyzed.

An ice storm is not quite rain and not quite snow. It freezes on impact, creating a magical and dangerous thick glaze on the earth's surface. Just getting around is risky. When I was in medical school in upstate New York, a minor ice storm knocked out our power for several days. The novelty of living by candlelight and on canned food quickly faded. When the lights turned back on in my apartment complex, I emerged a frazzled cavewoman. My white 1980s Ford Escort had transformed into a swan ice sculpture. To live under those conditions for six weeks, while pregnant or with children, is unimaginable.

Since it is unethical—and downright mean—to stress out a pregnant woman to test the physiological effects on her baby, cataclysmic events provide researchers with rare insight into the impact of prenatal maternal stress. As Dr. Szyf joked in a TED Talk, "God does experiments with humans called natural disasters."[12] Epidemiologists at McGill University in Quebec, led by Suzanne King, acted quickly to identify pregnant women exposed to the Great Canadian Ice Storm of 1998, or those who'd conceived around that time. As is typical with major storms, area hospitals reported a baby boom nine months later.

The McGill researchers identified 178 willing study participants. They collected blood and saliva samples to see if the disaster had imprinted itself on the women's bodies. The researchers checked the mothers' physiologic responses to stress, including cortisol levels, a hormone the body pumps out during stressful circumstances. They also collected data about the mothers' objective stress—such as the number of days without power. When the babies arrived, the research team followed the children's physical and behavioral development through age thirteen.

The researchers found that the ice storm babies born to the moms with the highest amount of objective stress had more behavioral, health, and language problems compared with the low- or moderate-objective stressed moms.[13] These children had higher-than-expected rates of asthma, autism, and metabolic and autoimmune disorders. The longer the lights stayed out, the greater the impact on the developing baby.[14] Much like the Dutch Famine, a mom's stressful experience affected her child before birth, leaving an environmental imprint that would stay with the baby for life.

Love or a famine or an ice storm doesn't directly change a child's DNA sequence, but epigenetic modifications allow for flexibility in adapting to an ever-changing world. These epigenetic changes have long-term consequences during critical developmental periods, but they also occur throughout our life span.

For Dr. Szyf and other scientists, one major question lingered: How do you know if methylation, or epigenetic change, isn't somehow caused by some other underlying unknown genetics? Could environment and life experience alone really alter genes? To find out, Dr. Szyf and his research team designed a study to look at the DNA of the Great Canadian Ice Storm babies as teenagers. Remember, this storm was an entirely random event; there was no chance to preprogram anything. Through careful analysis, the research team discovered that children of the most stressed moms showed a distinct pattern of DNA

The social environment modifies the story of a person's DNA.

methylation, particularly in immune and metabolic cells.[15] Their findings confirmed that genes didn't predetermine epigenetic changes: the social environment modifies the story of a person's DNA. And usually there is a reason.

Given the choice, a loving mother sounds greatly preferable to the alternative. So does a more nurturing womb. We perceive a lot of the epigenetic changes that come from distracted parenting or stressed pregnant mothers as negative, but we need to remember the flip side: they can help in certain situations. After all, epigenetic changes facilitate survival. A relaxed mother rat with time to lick her babies is lovely if she lives in a cage free from predators, whereas a relaxed rat in a world filled with cats is dinner. A low-licker rat mom's behavior can send an important early message for survival: "Baby Beware!" Anxiety, hypervigilance, and aggression improve survival when enemies lurk.

Similarly, a developing fetus adapts to urgent environmental needs for survival. The trade-off for initial survival may, however, mean trouble down the road. For instance, a baby born to a pregnant mom with poor nutrition may have epigenetic modifications to store extra fat when food is available. This adaptation is helpful for early survival, until he encounters a fast-food dollar menu.

The recognition that social experience alters DNA through epigenetics is a massive renaissance in science, medicine, and our most intimate relationships. Prior to the discovery of epigenetic processes, health was all about genetic determinism. Love and experience took a back seat. Until very recently, people thought the role of the parents wasn't that important in their children's lives. As Dr. Szyf explained, while he was raising his kids, most people believed that "if you were born with the right genes, you'd be fine." The genetics-as-everything view took the accountability off the parent. Dr. Szyf notes, "It was total freedom without blame." Oh, my. Cue the guilt.

And yet this scientific confirmation of the power of the child-parent bond will probably surprise few mothers or fathers. Studies of early development suggest living creatures have an innate drive to bond. Starting on the first day of life through thousands of tiny interactions with caregivers, a baby learns if the world is a safe and helpful place that will meet her needs. When the relationship is positive, and the child feels loved, the attachment is secure. Over time, strong attachments help children stay emotionally steady, bounce back from disappointment, and build friendships. She's likely to carry this attachment style into adulthood and eventually parenthood. As British developmental psychologist John Bowlby said, "All of us, from cradle to grave, are happiest when life is organized as a series of excursions, long or short, from the secure base provided by our attachment figures."

But as Bowlby knew from his work and personal life, things don't always go so smoothly. Insecure attachments result from absent, unreliable, abusive, or overbearing parent relationships. In the 1970s, Bowlby's star student and colleague, psychologist Mary Ainsworth, developed a test of attachment called the "strange situation." She studied what happened to children twelve to eighteen months old when a child was playing with her mom, and then a stranger entered the room. She also looked at what happened if the child's mother stepped out, and then how the child responded when she returned.[16]

A child under two with a secure attachment is friendly to the stranger when the mom is present, gets upset when Mom leaves, and is wary of the stranger when alone. She seems happy to see her mom on her return. Children with nonsecure attachments either show no distress when Mom leaves, seem okay with the stranger, and register little emotion when Mom returns (*avoidant attachment*); or show prolonged distress when Mom leaves, act fearful of the stranger, and become upset with the mom on her return, sometimes even pushing her away (*insecure attachment*). An extensive review of two thousand "strange situations" done in eight different countries shows insecure attachment present across cultures for about one out of every two kids.[17]

Decades of research since Bowlby and Ainsworth published their data shows that without intervention, insecure attachment as a kid translates into trouble expressing and regulating feelings as an adult. A person with a history of nonsecure attachment as a child may experience an intense fear of abandonment as a grown-up, and either avoid getting emotionally close to others or glom on to less-than-perfect partners and fall to pieces when things don't work out. Insecure attachment also leads to increased cortisol levels, lower hippocampal volume (an area of the brain involved in memory and learning), and greater risk of physical and mental illness.[18]

We know, in part, that children with secure attachments or relationships fare differently in life because of one of the longest-running studies in history. Starting at the end of the Great Depression in 1938, the Grant Study tracked a cohort of Harvard undergraduates, including the future president John F. Kennedy, into adulthood.[19] Over time the research expanded to participants' wives, children, and a comparison group of people from less affluent Boston neighborhoods. During the eight decades of research, principal investigator Dr. George Vaillant and his team consistently found one key predictor of a successful, healthy, happy life: good relationships.[20]

So if you're a parent, you know, no pressure.

Just thinking about attachment makes me want to run and hug my kids. From epigenetic research, we know a parent's love creates a cascade of positive health effects in her child. And even if we didn't grow up with a loving environment, we have an opportunity to foster one for ourselves and our children. This reminds me of a Steve Martin joke, "I gave my cat a bath the other day . . . they love it. He sat there, he enjoyed it, it was fun for me. The fur would stick to my tongue, but other than that . . ." So while we don't lick and groom our loved ones like a mama rat, there are ways our loving touch changes destiny.

For newborns, direct skin-on-skin contact is particularly critical. In those crucial moments following Jamie's birth, Kate Ogg instinctually placed her son on her bare skin, a practice known as "kangaroo care." When kangaroo babies are first born, they look like wiggly pink gummy bears. With no hair, they need the warmth of their mom's pouch to grow strong.

In 1978 neonatologist Dr. Edgar Rey Sanabria got a radical idea after reading an article about kangaroo babies' survival. He worked in Bogotá, Colombia, where three out of every four preterm infants receiving standard medical care in the hospital died. Out of desperation and overcrowded conditions, he asked new mothers to use their body heat as an incubator instead.[21] Given the number of babies dying, they had little to lose. The mother placed the child, in only a diaper, on her chest, making sure its nose and mouth were visible and unobstructed. Immediately Dr. Rey Sanabria noticed more babies survived.[22] Thousands of studies since have shown kangaroo care normalizes the baby's heart rate, breathing, and oxygen saturation. Down the road, these babies are calmer, sleep better, and have higher IQs. Around the world, often in countries with few resources, this practice reduces preterm infant mortality by over 30 percent.[23]

While the benefits of kangaroo care include physical warmth and the comforting sound of the parent's heartbeat, the neuropeptide oxytocin also plays a key role. Oxytocin is known as the "love hormone" because it's involved in bonding, empathy, and trust. It is released at childbirth and during breastfeeding, as well as when we hug, kiss, and snuggle. Oxytocin helps us remember faces and build connection, and it increases steadily during the first six months of parenting for both moms and dads.

Could love make us weak in the knees? While the hormone is produced in the brain and released via the pituitary gland into the bloodstream, receptors all over the body explain its widespread effects. Oxytocin helps us feel calm, appreciated, and even sing more. In one study of sixty-eight men, those who received a nasal oxytocin spray were 80 percent more generous sharing cash with a stranger than those who did not.[24] Babies are notoriously rude houseguests, so oxytocin helps. There's evidence that the hormone's released not just from kangaroo care and loving touch, but also with physical play, "raspberries" to the belly, peekaboo, surprise tickles, impersonating stuffed animals, and general silliness.

Kate Ogg's story of the seemingly miraculous recovery of her stillborn baby dramatically illustrates the healing power of physical warmth with our children. Yet touch is vital for every living creature throughout life. When we think about physical intimacy for adults, sex often comes to mind. And while sex plays a role, so too does casual physical touch in our everyday relationships. There is a biological reason that a friend's supportive hand on our shoulder or a pat on the back comforts us. Similar to the animal kingdom, social grooming is a part of social bonding. This might be why some women love their weekly salon blowouts and why we tend to stick with the same hairdresser over years.[25] In medicine, the comforting touch of your doctor, such as when using a stethoscope to listen to your heart and lungs, also might be part of why we stay loyal to the same physician over time.[26]

The sense of connection from touch is more than emotional attachment. There's also a physiological factor. Holding hands lowers blood pressure, heart rate, and cortisol.[27] Even twins in utero do it. One tender sonogram revealed one twin, who was healthy, and the other, who was gravely ill, holding hands in the womb.[28] Interlocking hands makes us feel brave. In the "lend a hand study," women who thought they were about to get an electric shock showed less threat activation on functional neuroimaging brain scans when they held the hand of their spouse or a stranger compared to not holding anyone's hand. (Holding a spouse's hand created the strongest response, but only if the marriage was healthy.)[29]

Studies show that when a person holds the hand of a loved one in distress, the breath and heartbeat of the pair sync up. Their bodies harmonize. Most amazing is that their brainwaves harmonize as well, which is known as entrainment. One study looked at twenty-two couples wearing brain wave monitors, or electroencephalography (EEG) caps, where one partner had heat placed on her arm for two minutes. Researchers found that the more empathetic her partner felt to her pain, the more in sync their brain waves. Additionally, the more synchronized the brain waves, the less pain she reported. Even being in the same room together but not touching, there was some "brain-to-brain" synchronization.[30] Similar to fireflies flashing in concert on a summer night.[31] A study in Nature's Scientific Reports shows when two people are talking and listening to each other, their brain oscillations synchronize beyond auditory processing alone.[32] They actually get on the same wavelength. Humans are emotionally and biologically connected in ways we don't fully understand, and touch is a key part of this.

Touch is also critical for health throughout the life span. Increasingly studies show the potential benefits of massage for preterm infants, children with autism, women with breast cancer, individuals with autoimmune disorders (including asthma and multiple sclerosis), and seniors with dementia.[33] A study of older adults showed that older patients who had a social visit and a brief massage have more cognitive and emotional benefits than those who just have a social visit alone.[34] In addition, it appears that the benefits of massage may extend not only to the receiver but to the giver as well.[35]

Hugs play a role in physical intimacy and health too. Researchers at Carnegie Mellon University examined the interplay between exposure to illness, social support, and daily hugs. In the name of science (and possibly a hundred bucks), 404 healthy adults agreed to inhale nasal drops that exposed them to the common cold. First, the researchers drew blood samples to confirm that the volunteers were not immune. Then they surveyed the participants over fourteen consecutive days, asking about disagreements and hugs received. Finally, they exposed volunteers to the cold virus and monitored symptoms, such as mucus production, in quarantine for five days. Those who got daily hugs were 32 percent less likely to get sick.[36]

Hugs don't make you impervious to a cold, it turns out. But the huggers who did get sick didn't get *as* sick. They had less severe symptoms and got better faster. The more hugs, the better, yes. But just one a day seemed to make a difference. When my youngest son, Zay, was three, we went around the dinner table on December 31 asking about New Year's resolutions or goals for the next year. He announced his was to "give more hugs." Turns out, he might have been onto something. Ideal hug length seems to be between six and twenty seconds, which is a bit longer than most of us are used to.[37] In America, enough people feel starved for physical contact that there is increasing demand for paid platonic cuddler services, along with professional snuggler certifications and conventions (such as Cuddle Con). These services seem more legit than that smiley guy at the park holding a "free hugs" sign.

Touch isn't the only way we establish intimate bonds. Simply paying attention to our loved ones also matters. At Columbia University's Vagelos College of Physicians and Surgeons, first-year medical students watch a video of normal child development. The video shows a mom and her baby, sitting facing each other. They are happily interacting. Smiles and delighted coos go back and forth. It's charming. Next, the mom's face suddenly falls flat, and she becomes unresponsive to the child's attempts at interaction. She turns away. The baby tries to reengage her with coos, to no avail. The baby becomes visibly distraught and cries out. Eventually, with no response, the baby looks away too. It is painful to watch. When normal interaction resumes, there is temporary relief, but things are not quite what they were before. The child looks uncertain and upset.

Numerous follow-up studies show the robustness of the "still-face effect" where, after the parent reengages, the child smiles less and looks sideways more. Tests using a novel environmental cue show that babies seem to recall this upsetting episode a couple of weeks later. Child development researcher Edward Tronick and his colleagues designed the still-face experiment in the 1970s, well before the discovery of reflexive mirroring in developing empathy. Research from neuroscience indicates that we unknowingly and automatically are wired to mimic the facial expressions of the people we interact with during the day.[38] This mirroring helps children develop empathy, which we will discuss more in chapter 8. But you have to be looking at a person for this to happen, and paying attention in a distracted world is easier said than done.

Tronick's study was also well before we inadvertently started doing the still-face experiment with our children multiple times a day while looking at our smartphones. At a conference on mindfulness in New York City, Arianna Huffington asked the audience, "What's your relationship with your phone? Are you sleeping together?" I could barely look up from my screen to consider the question. Our eldest son, Max, was born around the advent of the iPhone, and time spent coddling our new device undoubtedly eclipsed time spent snuggling our new son. We are in an unchartered relationship with technology, and so are our children. This much is clear: Your child will grow up to be a different person if you pay attention and lock eyes with them more. And if you don't, you may be unconsciously reshaping their genetic scripts in ways that will affect your grandchildren and great-grandchildren. Suddenly it seems that email can wait.

The presence or absence of close bonds, the first ring of the hidden factors, can literally have life-changing impact. Not just for babies like Kate Ogg's, but also for couples, for whom marriage is so closely tied to health. For example, Esther Klein and George Szekeres met as university students in 1933 in Budapest. At a casual meet up, along with their good friend Paul Erdős (whom we'll discuss in chapter 5), Esther proposed a challenging geometry problem that she was working on and George eventually helped solve. After the couple fell in love and married in 1937, the puzzle subsequently became known as the "happy ending problem." But the times were changing in Hungary, and with the uncertain political atmosphere, a happy ending was no guarantee.

To escape Nazi persecution, the couple relocated to Shanghai, China, in 1939. There, George found work as a leather chemist, and the couple eventually found themselves caught up in the Japanese occupation and brewing Communist revolution.[39] To escape turmoil again, in 1948 George accepted a mathematics position at a university in Australia. With the intellectual freedom to reengage with academics, the pair became two of the most influential mathematicians of the twentieth century. After two children and nearly seventy years of marriage, their remarkable journey wasn't over yet. Side by side in the same nursing home room, the couple died of natural causes within thirty minutes of each other. Esther and George Szekeres's intimate bond carried them through an incredibly eventful, stressful, and joyful life. In a very different way, that bond carried them through death as well.[40]

Our intimate, one-on-one bonds are the most important critical hidden factor in our health. From the earliest moments of life, they are the building blocks of trust and attachment that can carry us through a lifetime of relationships. Strong one-on-one bonds also provide us with a solid base to navigate our world and peacefully manage conflicts that arise, as we will discuss in chapter 10. And as adults, there are healthy steps we can take to boost our intimate connections (see the tool kit box on page 31).

> **Our intimate, one-on-one bonds are the most important critical hidden factor in our health.**

Collectively, we can also help others form healthy connections in their families during critical times. In 2018 only two countries in the whole world didn't mandate paid maternity leave: Papua New Guinea and the United States of America. Meanwhile, data shows that ten weeks of paid parental leave reduces infant mortality by 10 percent. It also helps a child be more likely to see her fifth birthday, possibly because of more time for breastfeeding.[41] Kate and Jamie's story moves us. Together, through better maternity policies, we can save even more Jamies.

The exciting field of epigenetics shows a mother's love and intimacy with her child shapes DNA in ways medicine is just beginning to understand. As Dr. Szyf observes, this makes genetics like an interactive movie. Just as the Oggs did with Jamie, we have the power to rewrite the script. We can transform an initially shaky bond into one that bolsters health and well-being. As Dr. Szyf explains, "Whether 5 percent or 95 percent of the script is predetermined, it doesn't matter." It's easy to hear the excitement in his voice as he says, "That's huge!" Even if we had a messed-up childhood and are in an unhappy

> Data shows that ten weeks of paid parental leave reduces infant mortality by 10 percent.

marriage, epigenetics offers us the hope of change for the future. Genetics don't determine our destiny; we do. Or as my ten-year-old son, Max, told me in the wise way children have, "The most important thing in life is love." Our intimate relationships are a key part of that. So, too, are our relationships with our friends, colleagues, and neighbors, as we'll explore next.

EXPAND YOUR TOOL KIT

One-on-One Relationships

Consider your closest intimate relationships. What aspects, either past or present, have you enjoyed the most? What elements might you consider expanding in new or more intentional ways? Here are some ideas to get you started in the process of discovering what feels authentic and works for you.

> Express your love for family, children, and grandchildren in a way that feels comfortable to you. For some this may be physical or nonphysical affection, such as sharing words, food, a helping hand, or anticipating needs.

> Ways to increase comforting touch with those you love in your life may include more hugs, hand-holding, smooches, and snuggles. If it's an option, pop on a movie or read a book and cuddle on the couch. Offer a teen a pat on the back, shoulder squeeze, or high five when you greet. It may be something you have to consciously think about at first, but it's a rewarding bonding process.

> If you live alone, add touch to your life in other ways: chair massages, hair blowouts, mani/pedis, get your makeup done, or a foot/hand rub. While self-care may sound like a luxury, touch is absolutely critical for every human being.

> Lock eyes more with those you love. Try to hold their gaze for longer than feels comfortable. If you have small children in your life, challenge them to a staring contest, or mimic one another's silly faces.

> Full attention may require that everyone puts their phone away or on airplane mode during family time. Cut down on

activities that distract you from paying full attention. Can that email (news, TV show) wait? Can you check emails just during work hours? Spend less time posting on social media and more time actually being social. Try an old-fashioned board game night. Play cards and practice your best poker face and playful trash talk. Or on your next family outing, pretend you're living in a pre-smartphone world. Consider using an instant camera instead of using a phone for pictures. Please don't let moments with the ones you love pass you by.

> Before you pick something at random off your friends' baby registry, support new moms and dads in a way that gives them more time with their little one. Drop off a tray of frozen homemade lasagna, offer to run errands or take the older children out for a day, or pay for a laundry or housekeeper service.

> Good relationships are the most important ingredient in a happy, healthy, successful life, so invest your time accordingly. Set boundaries around work hours to protect family time and commitments. Schedule a few hours each week (literally put them on your schedule) to check in with those you love. Put love and connection first. Model this for your kids. Make a point of giving your kids, spouse, or dog a hug, kiss, or high five walking out the door in the morning. You just never know what a day holds.

> Celebrate your history. Consider a "they grow up so fast" family night to show your child or grandchild old photos or videos from when she was little. Show her old family photos and tell the stories that go with them. (This is also fun to do with your longtime friends.) If you are married, for your anniversary, get all dressed up and watch your old wedding footage. Break out the bubbly and make a toast.

‣ To boost oxytocin and mood, lighten up. Be sillier. Smell the roses. Take a dance class at the YMCA (I recently started hip-hop) or turn on a portable disco light (I got one for twenty dollars online) and dance your heart out. It's hard to stay in a bad mood while you're doing "the snake." Laugh when your neighbors see you. You get the idea.

‣ Just as you want to raise your heart rate in exercise, you want to find activities that fill your heart with love so that you can share it with others. So please take time for yourself too.

Chapter Three

Social Ties: Your Community

A faithful friend is the medicine of life.
—ECCLESIASTES PROVERB

On Okinawa Island, two hours by plane south of mainland Japan, there are more people over the age of one hundred than anywhere else in the world. The longevity has taken on an almost mystical appeal. Visitors who come to see the island's aqua blue waters could nearly forget Okinawa's decimation in World War II. The Battle of Okinawa that took place on Easter Sunday in 1945 was known as the "typhoon of steel" and left the island with half its original population. While one may wonder if the postwar longevity is a cruel Darwinian survival of the fittest, Okinawa's reputation for long life predates the 1940s. Its longtime nickname among Asian neighbors is "the Land of the Immortals."

No one could figure out what contributed to the Okinawans' longevity. Health researchers have long searched the Okinawan diet for clues to the fountain of youth. Perhaps the key lay in a unique compound in the tea, or mugwort, or *goya*? What kind of seaweed do the island's residents consume? Scientists have pursued similar scientific dietary explorations in other cultures known for longevity, such as in the Mediterranean.

The thinking is, *If only we could decode the perfect combination of foods from around the world and put the vital nutrients in a pill, we could live long enough to chase around our great-grandchildren*. But what if we're looking for answers in the wrong places?

Some clues to what the Okinawans get right may lie in a study, far from Okinawa, involving Roseto, a small town in northeastern Pennsylvania just south of Bear Swamp and Lake Minge and about two hours west of New York City. In 1961 a physician from this small, predominantly Italian American community met Dr. Stewart Wolf, a physician and public health researcher at the University of Oklahoma, for a beer after a medical conference. The physician from Roseto claimed that the patients he saw there over the previous decade weren't dying of heart disease like the rest of the country. He reported that he'd never seen anyone under the age of fifty-five with a heart attack. There were no suicides or peptic ulcer disease either. It seemed to him the citizens of Roseto weren't really dying of anything but old age.

Back home in Oklahoma, Dr. Wolf kept thinking about Roseto. At the time, the leading cause of death in the nation among middle-aged men was heart disease. Dr. Wolf verified that Roseto residents did have far fewer heart attacks than other US or even Italian American communities. Dr. Wolf learned that the town's overall yearly death rate, one death per thousand people, was about 50 percent less than in neighboring towns, such as Bangor or Nazareth. It was as if the people of Roseto, Pennsylvania, had never left rural Italy.

Curious to learn more, he mobilized a research team to go to Roseto. With the support of the town mayor, the investigators went house to house, knocking on doors. They evaluated 86 percent of the population in just four weeks. The team constructed family histories, performed physicals, and did EKGs. They culled through death certificates and medical records. No clinic's filing cabinet was left unexamined on the quest for the Holy Grail of Roseto's good health. The researchers considered diet, alcohol consumption, smoking, exercise, and genetics. What was remarkable is how unremarkable all those things were. People in Roseto enjoyed stogies, sausages, and loafing around as much as people in nearby towns. They worked dangerous jobs in quarries, cooked with lard, and were more overweight than expected. If anything, their diet and lifestyle should've knocked years off their life. No clear biological explanation accounted for the physiologic advantage.

Confused, the researchers looked up from their graph paper and slide rules. The team considered Roseto itself. Only then did they appreciate the unique social landscape. As they shuttled between hospitals and clinics, in the community people were chatting on the street, friends sat on porches, toddlers played with grandparents, and multigenerational families shared meals. Families with money didn't flaunt it. Neighbors supported one another in hard times. A distinct sense of belonging, trust, and equality permeated the community. During the early 1960s, the reported crime rate was nearly zero. Dr. Wolf and his colleagues, including medical sociologist Dr. John Bruhn, hypothesized that what was remarkable about Roseto was its close-knit social ties.[1] They also knew time would tell. As Bob Dylan famously predicted in his 1964 song, "The times they are a-changin.'"

After 1965 daily life in America started to shift. Reports found that in the United States, people felt more disconnected from one another. As Harvard political scientist Robert Putnam wrote in his seminal book they began "bowling alone."[2] Participation in dinner clubs, social groups, and other community events after work slowed. People had Technicolor television to watch. Young go-getters in small towns left for brighter prospects in bigger cities. Class differences became more apparent with country club memberships, swanky cars, and travel to far-off places like Hawaii. Roseto was no exception.

The sense of community and egalitarianism that had defined Roseto faded. In 1971, for the first time in the town's history, a person under the age of forty-five died from a heart attack. Researchers continued to watch and collect data. A thirty-year follow-up study showed that heart attack rates in Roseto gradually rose to match that of neighboring town Bangor.[3] The long-term findings confirmed that the original "Roseto effect" was a perfect example of the importance of positive social connections in health.

If social ties explain the Roseto effect and its subsequent disappearance, might they also be the hidden factor in health that can explain Okinawa's immortals? Let's return to our Japanese centenarians for a closer look. Though many researchers focus on what the Okinawans eat, figuring out the secret to a long life span may require looking up from the plate.

While diet plays a role in health, my Mediterranean take-out is a fairly lonely affair. There is little laughter or sense of community while I wait in line to buy my lunch; I don't share stories of my day with the guy behind the counter as he prepares it. If I did, I might get a strange look. Downing my food in front of my computer, I don't achieve a sense of deep relaxation or well-being. My meal occurs in isolation.

In places like Japan, Italy, Greece, and France, by contrast, meals are a highly social occasion. The preparation is social and often multigenerational. It is a major activity of the day. Kids sit side by side with family and guests. It's not just *what* one is eating, but with *whom* one is eating. Meals under the Tuscan sun are savored with friends and family.

In Okinawa, sharing isn't restricted to meals. Okinawans get together often. They celebrate birthdays and anniversaries as a group. They participate in *moai*, or gatherings for a common purpose. They laugh a lot. Centenarians on Okinawa belong to pop bands, practice karate, eat dinner with their great-grandchildren, and celebrate *ikigai*, or their sense of a life well lived.[4] An Okinawan is socially connected, and not just in a Facebook or Twitter kind of way.

In short, Okinawans take care of one another. For example, in an island program, seniors care for super-seniors (the oldest old) for several hours a day. It's an engaging social experience for both age brackets and a sharp contrast to the isolating nursing home experience of most older Americans. In Okinawa and other places where people live exceptionally long lives, public health research suggests it isn't the diet but the community in which the meals occur that makes all the difference.

As a kid, my mom and I read *The Secret Garden* by Frances Hodgson Burnett together. I loved the children's secret life and Mary's ingenuity. While it remains one of my favorite children's fiction books, I now understand the story through a different lens. After her parents die, ten-year-old Mary gets sent off to live with an uncle she has never met in a vast and lonely manor in England. At night she hears mysterious screams, which she eventually discovers belong to her sickly cousin, Colin. For his safety, Colin is confined to a sterile room in the home, where he's withered away and become too weak to walk. His father, Lord Craven, cannot bear to see his son suffering and departs for far-off lands. Mary, not one for rules, stages a prison break to show Colin a secret garden that she has discovered on the property and tended with another boy. With repeated visits to the garden, surrounded by fresh air, laughter, and friends, Colin regains his strength. So, too, does Mary. Even the glum Lord Craven, on his return to the manor, is uplifted by the children's joy. The story perfectly exemplifies the importance of social ties for good health—and how social isolation is the surprise villain.

Social ties are a critical hidden factor of health, yet we often pay more attention to our diet and devices than to our communities. Despite all our technology, social disconnection in America remains a serious problem. In the US, around one in five adults report chronic loneliness and some studies suggest that number is on the rise.[5] Among people over sixty, more than 40 percent report feeling lonely.[6] UK Researchers found in 2015 that one in four people over seventy-five goes days without seeing or talking to anyone, and for about 40 percent of older adults, their primary companion is the TV.[7] Younger people may not fare much better: one in ten kids say they don't have any friends.[8] Isolation seems particularly problematic for boys, who are nearly twice as likely to report having no close confidants.[9] As Professor John Cacioppo at the University of Chicago describes, "Loneliness isn't about being alone; it's about not feeling connected."[10]

Social relationships are defined both by quantity and quality. It helps explain Elvis Presley feeling lonely in a crowded room.[11] Loneliness has two components. It's *objective*—the number of people who live in your home, the distance between you and your family and friends, and how often you interact and get together with people. It's also *subjective*, meaning it can leave us feeling left out or isolated. Tolstoy begins *Anna Karenina* with, "Happy families are all alike; every unhappy family is unhappy in its own way." And loneliness is one of those ways—even when you're sleeping next to someone. Marriage is protective, but only for the happily married.[12] My work in mental health has shown me that when you pull back the curtain on money or fame, everyone feels lonely at times.

Loneliness is like the killer lurking in the basement in a horror movie. In short bursts, up to a few days at a time, it motivates us to reconnect with others. When loneliness is prolonged, it's riskier than well-established hazards such as obesity, physical inactivity, high blood pressure, and bad cholesterol.[13] In a meta-analysis that looked at the health of nearly 4 million people, obesity increased the risk of an early death by 30 percent, whereas loneliness increased it by 50 percent.[14] We talk about the obesity epidemic, but what about the millions of lonely people? Feeling chronically lonely increases the odds of heart disease and stroke by about 30 percent.[15] Loneliness is equivalent to smoking fifteen cigarettes a day or heavy alcohol use.[16]

> **Loneliness is equivalent to smoking fifteen cigarettes a day or heavy alcohol use.**

Social isolation can develop into a self-fulfilling prophecy known as the "loneliness loop." Rory got caught in it. He was a quiet twenty-six-year-old man who spoke with a soft Texas drawl. Always an introvert, he'd left his small town for an opportunity he couldn't pass up in the Big Apple. Several months into his new life in New York City, he still felt like a fish out of water. Shortly after he'd arrived, he went to dinner at a hip downtown restaurant with coworkers from his new tech company. Right after his salad came, Rory suddenly became short of breath with a pounding heart. In the moment, he felt afraid he was dying. He got up suddenly from the candlelit table and smashed a full wineglass to the floor in the process. He explained, "The whole place stopped and stared at me." He went to the ER, convinced he was having a heart attack. Several hours later, he learned his heart was fine. "Just a panic attack," the doctor said.

But after that, he felt embarrassed and said no to after-hours events with coworkers. Eventually, they stopped asking. Not knowing a lot of people, it was easy to sit on his couch and binge watch his favorite series on TV. The less he engaged, the less he was invited, and the worse he felt about himself. He hadn't gone out on a date since he arrived. His family back home had no idea how bad things had gotten. He didn't want to worry them.

Rory was in deep. Avoidance of others lowers self-esteem and creates pessimism that perpetuates the loneliness loop. A person who feels rejected or isolated acts stressed, fearful, and hypervigilant, like someone in physical danger. This is a true physiological response. After all, neuroimaging studies show the brain processes social rejection and physical pain similarly.[17] Feeling like you've been stabbed in the back is closer to actually being stabbed in the back than you'd think. Brain studies of people after unwanted breakups show that rejection hurts, physically.[18] As living creatures, we instinctively avoid pain. And like Daisy, our patient from chapter 1 who felt sick but appeared well on all diagnostic tests, loneliness takes a hidden physical toll.

Study after study shows the impact social ties can have on our health. I learned in medical school that increased exposure to an infectious disease increased the risk of getting the disease. It sounds logical. One would think the more people you come into contact with, the more risk of exposure to germs, and the higher odds of getting sick. This understanding of disease was the basis for programs at the turn of the twentieth century in countries around the world where officials forcibly removed children from their homes and put them in institutions to avoid potential tuberculosis exposure.[19] But we now know it's just not that simple. Similar to how a hug can build our resistance to the common cold, evidence suggests that a person with a more extensive social circle is more *protected* from infection.[20] It's difficult to reconcile the data on social support with the germ theory of disease. It doesn't fit the current biomedical model in its skintight form. But this isn't hot-off-the-press research. The studies go back decades.

In the 1940s orphanages in Austria had a very high death rate—about one out of three kids died. To lose this many kids horrified Dr. René Spitz. At the time doctors blamed contagious diseases for the high death rate, so children were kept in isolated cribs away from one another. Yet Dr. Spitz noticed children on pediatric wards in incubators did worse than those whose parents couldn't afford such state-of-the-art care and who were held by nurses instead. This was decades before Dr. Nerem conducted the rabbit studies in the 1970s, but Dr. Spitz had a hunch that the love of those nurses protected their charges' health. After all, humans are innately social creatures. Dr. Spitz worried that the orphanages that tried to create a sterile environment harmed children by emotional deprivation.[21]

To study if his theory was correct, Dr. Spitz followed two groups of kids during their first years of life. Group one consisted of babies living in the sterile conditions of an orphanage. The second group of babies lived in a prison nursery near their mothers. Doctors believed the children at the prison were at high risk of death from overcrowding and disease. But Dr. Spitz found the exact opposite. Children raised in the isolation of the orphanage showed more developmental problems, such as delayed walking and talking, and suffered far more infections.[22] During the study, three to four out of every ten children in the orphanage died and none of those who lived in the prison died.[23] None. Love and connection triumphed, as they often quietly do, but the practice did not change.

In 2007 orphaned children in Bucharest, Romania, were still being raised in relative isolation. Researchers again challenged the status quo, this time in a randomized controlled trial that was published in *Science*.[24] They looked at two groups of abandoned children over the course of four and a half years. One set of children were raised in institutions like orphanages, and the second started life in institutions before transitioning into foster care (about 46 percent of foster families were single mothers). In 2007 the institutions remained the gold standard of care in Romania, and the government held that there was no benefit to foster care. The researchers studied only healthy children, so critics couldn't argue that the institutionalized children were a sicker group to begin with. Sixty years later, Dr. Spitz's original findings held up: the kids placed with foster families had significant health advantages, from growth and attention to cognitive abilities and behavior, over the kids in the institutions. The earlier and younger the child got moved from the institution into foster care, the better the outcome. Two conclusive studies later, one would hope that we would understand that separating and institutionalizing children is inhumane.[25]

A prospective study from New Zealand offers clues to how loneliness erodes health starting in childhood. Researchers interested in the effects of social isolation followed over a thousand kids starting at birth. Initially, the researchers asked the children's teachers standardized questions about their students' social functioning. Then, when the kids reached their teens, the researchers asked the children directly whether they felt alone even with friends or if other people were worried about their well-being. The researchers controlled for other factors such as family income, low IQ, and being overweight.

Twenty-six years later, the study published in *JAMA*'s *Archives* series revealed that socially isolated children have worse health. As young adults they had a 37 percent increased risk of cardiovascular disease, including being overweight and having elevated blood pressure, and other metabolic issues. There was a clear dose-response, meaning the more isolated the child, the greater the negative effect.[26] (A dose-response is a research finding that gets epidemiologists to sit on the edge of their chairs with excitement and is considered robust evidence for a causal relationship.)

In a follow-up study of the socially isolated children, when the group turned thirty-two years old, those who had experienced childhood isolation had an 87 percent increased risk of developing age-related diseases in adulthood, including higher rates of major depression, inflammation, obesity, high blood pressure, high cholesterol, and metabolic disturbances.[27] An epidemiologist just fell off her chair.

The data seems crystal clear: it's time to take socializing as seriously as exercise, diet, and sleep. Study after study builds on the mounting pile of evidence that social support in our community is necessary for wellness. Laughter, warmth, respect, trust, caring, and support are good for physical health. Research from Oxford professor of evolutionary psychology Dr. Robin Dunbar indicates three, four, or five close friends are optimal for health; however, even just one person who has your back helps.[28]

A close-knit community like Roseto or Okinawa offers its residents a safety net. Our social ties buffer us physically and mentally. With friends or family on your side, a crappy situation makes for a good story later. Supportive relationships allow you to brush off an uncivil coworker, a lousy date, that creep on the subway, and various iterations of bullies. After something terrible happens, it's easy to toss and turn at night. Better social support improves sleep quality, which improves cognitive functioning and mood.[29] Good relationships reduce blood pressure, inflammation, and the fight-or-flight hormones epinephrine and cortisol.[30] Supportive relationships also increase oxytocin, the "love hormone," and endogenous opioids, reducing pain.[31] Altogether, knowing that others have your back offsets the impact of stress on the body. In Okinawa, strong friendships and community likely buffered the devastation and horror of World War II.

A 1988 meta-analysis in *Science* called "Social Relationships and Health," which other researchers have cited more than 6,500 times, was the first of its kind to summarize swaths of data showing that people with better relationships live longer.[32] Since that article was published over thirty years ago, countless additional studies have backed up its findings. In 2010 Dr. Julianne Holt-Lunstad and her colleagues at Brigham Young University reviewed 148 studies, with a total of 308,849 participants. The researchers found people with active social circles had a 50 percent increased likelihood of survival compared to people with weaker social relationships. Age, gender, or even other medical problems weren't a factor. The researchers controlled for those. The difference in mortality risk came down to one key thing: positive connections with others.[33] People who scored high on measures of more complex social integration (such as marital status, number of friends, and involvement with friends) got the biggest survival boost. If this came in a pill, I'd take it every day. But it turns out I don't have to. I can just grab brunch.

Volunteering, visiting Great-Aunt Polly, attending book clubs, every bit of positive connection helps. Belly laughs with friends correlate with improved heart health, circulation, and decreased pain perception. Social butterflies catch fewer colds.[34] Women with active friendships have healthier hearts, stronger immune systems, and less anxiety and depression.[35] College students with strong social networks show a more robust response to the flu vaccine compared to students with smaller social networks, thus improving the vaccine's effectiveness.[36] If you have extra time to give, studies show that spending as little as one hour a month delivering meals to homebound individuals not only boosts mood and well-being for everyone involved, but helps the volunteer live longer too.[37]

Maybe if you volunteer, a friend of yours is more likely to volunteer too. It turns out that good habits can pass from one person to another almost like a contagious illness. Dr. Nicholas Christakis and Dr. James Fowler demonstrated this using a massive set of data called the Framingham Heart Study database. The study has tracked numerous aspects of more than five thousand people's lives in Framingham, Massachusetts, since 1948.[38] Christakis and Fowler's "friend of a friend" research shows social factors, such as happiness, altruism, loneliness, smoking, and obesity spread through social ties.[39] Graphs show they also "cluster" within up to three degrees of separation.[40] In other words, the waistline of a friend of a friend helps predict mine. This evidence implies that what happens to someone loosely connected to me unknowingly impacts me both mentally and physically, and my behavior affects her.

Social contagion defies biomedicine's understanding of illness. But how does it work? Potential mechanisms include the "I'll have what she's having" effect (*direct impact*) versus the "birds of a feather" phenomenon (*homophily*). The direct impact theory of social contagion is that we consciously change our health behavior based on social connections, even weak ones. For instance, in line at a coffee shop, I grabbed a green vegetable juice. The woman behind me said, "I was going to have a latte, but you inspired me," and grabbed a green juice too. In a less healthy example, if you go out to lunch and your friend orders a cheeseburger, you may be tempted to order one, too, even though you'd originally planned to have a salad. Similarly, you are far more likely to show up to the gym when your friend is there waiting to work out with you. Positive (and negative) health behaviors of our companions over time nudge us toward protective (or harmful) behaviors with related epigenetic, cardiovascular, immune, and endocrine changes. This is known as the direct impact.

Alternatively, it could just be that we unconsciously find friends like us, aka birds of a feather. Maybe people who work out regularly or eat vegan are friends to begin with or hang out in the same cafés. Curious similarities appear when examining the DNA of close friends; people seem to befriend individuals with similar genes. To check for homophily, Christakis and Fowler looked at friends of almost two thousand participants in the Framingham data set, where most people are of European ancestry. They compared the genes of friends to those of strangers. After looking at millions of genetic variations, they found good friends turned out to be the genetic equivalent of about fourth cousins. In particular, these friends seemed to have the most similarity in the genes coding for smell.[41] Since doing a DNA analysis over brunch or after work drinks is unlikely, it is not clear how someone unknowingly communicates her genes to a potential friend or mate. Genetic evidence suggests it's not just looks or skin color.

Other theories to explain the mysterious likenesses of friends include pheromones, or tiny airborne hormones, passing unconscious messages to others. After all, animals use pheromones to communicate. This invisible chemistry may explain why you "click" with one person and not another. Research by Dr. Martha McClintock and colleagues shows a person's preference for different humans' smells may be based on immune markers.[42] Precisely how social contagion happens is not entirely clear, but its effects are evident at the group level. And when you are part of a circle of friends with healthy habits, the contagion is a plus: everyone gets healthier.

Social relationships are also a significant predictor of decreased morbidity, meaning not just living longer, but better. When people do get sick, social supports offset the severity of the illness. A good example of this is Bella, who, despite her pancreatic cancer diagnosis, still bakes cowgirl cookies with her neighbors. Clinically speaking, this means less intense and fewer symptoms and better day-to-day functioning even among people with severe diseases, such as cancers, autoimmune diseases, or infections. Similarly, engagement in many social spheres, from friend to relative to spouse to community, improves lung functioning for older adults.[43]

Social support also keeps dementia at bay. A prospective study followed seniors (the average age at the start of the study was about eighty) for up to twelve years. No one had dementia at the beginning of the study. The researchers found that seniors who participated in community activities, attended sporting events, went out to dinner with family or friends, or attended church had a 70 percent decreased risk of dementia. Every extra social activity or interaction seemed to bring with it a significant cognitive boost.[44] Given these dramatic results, maybe health insurance shouldn't just cover medications for seniors but discount season basketball tickets.

As individuals going about our day-to-day lives, it's easy to forget that we're actors in an extensive network. Every person on the planet is enmeshed in the vibrant social network influencing our collective health and beliefs. The sum of a social network is far greater than its parts, yet the parts can influence the whole.

In 1988, after years traveling abroad, François Pasquier returned home to France to host a get-together for friends with the idea "Bring a meal, and bring a new friend." The dinner party was too big for his place, so he asked everyone to meet in a public spot for a picnic under the stars. He also requested that everyone dress in white so they could find one another. Fast-forward thirty years, and Dîner en Blanc has ten thousand "friends of friends" attending. Everyone brings their own tables, plates, food, decorations, champagne, and garbage bags for cleanup. The location is undisclosed until a couple of hours beforehand to add to the fun. It has inspired other inclusive pop-up picnics around the globe. In 2011 Garrett Sathre and Nicole Benjamin-Sathre posted an idea for a similar dinner in San Francisco's Golden Gate Park on a Facebook page, and 3,500 people showed up.[45] They now organize the dinners, often for charity, around the country.

Another example of bringing people together involves the inspiring story of a young woman named Lili Rachel Smith. Lili was born with Apert syndrome, which prematurely fuses the bones of the skull, changing the shape of the face. The craniofacial syndrome often requires numerous childhood surgeries. Lili handled many challenges, including social isolation, with charisma and courage. In middle school, though she was not bullied or teased, Lili felt invisible. At lunchtime, uncertain what to do after eating alone, she'd retreat to a toilet stall and call her mom. Social isolation, as many adolescents know, too often becomes insidious, and it is heartbreaking for parents to watch. Through Lili's activism for social justice and human rights, she eventually made many friends, and ultimately, her life and story helped spark a national movement to change the culture of middle school.[46]

At age fifteen, Lili died unexpectedly in her sleep of natural causes relating to her condition. After her tragic passing, her friends asked her mom, Laura Talmus, what they might do to help. Together, they founded the student-led organization called Beyond Differences.[47] Laura, who serves as the executive director, explained to me, "We envision a world where every child is accepted, valued, and included by their peers no matter what their differences." The organization is the only one singularly focused on ending youth isolation and has several national initiatives for middle schoolers, including No One Eats Alone (NOEA) Day.[48] The premise for the annual event (held every February around Valentine's Day in all fifty states) is simple: Make sure no one sits alone at lunch. Make it an expectation to ask people you don't usually sit with, and new classmates, to join you. Laura explains, "We inspire students themselves in all middle schools nationwide to end social isolation and create a culture of belonging for everyone."[49]

I experienced NOEA Day firsthand at PS 278 in New York City, along with 180 sixth through eighth graders. The event was organized by educator Raisa Sterling and a dozen extraordinary student leaders. "Miss Sterling," as the kids call her, exudes the warmth and strength of a teacher who does not give up on any student. As I observed the assembly and then lunch, I remembered two things. First, the incredible volume of middle school chatter: At times, teachers needed to use an actual megaphone. And second, in that cacophony, how challenging it can feel to know your voice matters. Even decades later entering the school cafeteria, I felt the tug of loneliness from when I was the new kid in eighth grade in Reno, Nevada, trying to figure out where to sit at lunch. At NOEA Day listening to the students bravely share stories of times they felt isolated, I realized how much this was something I needed when I was in their shoes. There is great comfort in knowing you're not alone.

Companionship is critical across the life span. It can also come with four fuzzy feet. Studies show that a loving pet reduces blood pressure, heart disease, and stress.[50] Pets boost mood, keep people out of the doctor's office, and help people live longer with abnormal heart rhythms or after a heart attack. A large Swedish study published in *Nature* in 2017 found that dog ownership for single-person households is associated with a significantly lower risk of heart disease (11 percent reduced risk) and all-cause death (33 percent reduced risk).[51] Nearly every pet owner (93 percent) says their furry friend makes them "a better person," such as more patient, responsible, and affectionate.[52] And another poll found one out of three people prefer their pets to their partners.[53] Perhaps it's the look of unconditional love Sir Winston Fur-chill offers while your partner cringes as you sing off-key in your underwear. It seems positive social relationships of all walks help us live longer and better.

Starting out as a doctor, I'd have never guessed that building strong positive relationships is not just fun, but an essential component of health. In the simple act of showing up, an individual has more sway than she may realize. As we continue through the rings, we'll look at our next circle of influence where we foster social connection and community: work. Social ties make a dramatic difference to our health, and combined with our jobs, also play a significant role in our day-to-day well-being.

EXPAND YOUR TOOL KIT

Social Ties

Take a moment to think about your friends and people you like spending time with. What aspects do you enjoy the most? What activities might you consider doing more of? How could you deepen your connections and expand your social circle? Here are some ideas to pick and choose from to find what is practical and fun for you.

› Make meals a social occasion. At home, if you live with others, carve out the time to hang out during preparation and eating. Invite a friend or family over, even when your home isn't totally immaculate—they won't care. (Perfection is overrated.) If, like me, you don't cook, host a potluck, or order takeout. See if you can make dinner a festive gathering for no reason—even if it means ordering a pizza on a random Tuesday night.

› If you are a teacher or parent, consider bringing No One Eats Alone Day (the program for middle school students inspired by Lili Smith) to your school. Check out www.nooneeatsalone.org and request a free backpack full of materials to launch your own event. Also check out www.beyonddifferences.org for more inspiring programs about how to create a culture of belonging and end youth isolation.

› Nurture your friendships. Make a point to show up to celebrate or acknowledge important events in your friends' lives. Send a quick note to or call people you haven't talked to in a while, just to let them know you're thinking about them. If a friend lives far away, plan a weekend get-together. Start a group text for your school pals who live in different cities and organize a retreat or conference call to catch up. Consider how you might connect friends with similar interests to build their social circles too. The more, the merrier.

> Plant new seeds. A way to meet new people is to join a local club, take a class (i.e., language classes are often free at the local library), or find an interest group. If you're feeling adventurous, consider saving for a trip somewhere you have always wanted to visit. For example, various women-only tours cater to solo travelers of all ages.

> If you're shy, or find that social situations give you anxiety, invite people you want to get to know better to meet you for an activity with a clear focus (i.e., a movie, play, museum tour, park cleanup, lecture, trivia night, concert, library event, yoga class, or book club). That way there is less pressure to generate conversation. Expect to hear some "no thanks" to your invitations. Leave the door open. While it may be disappointing, declined invitations let you know you're trying hard enough and casting a wide enough net. Go you!

> Consider hanging out with friends who make you laugh a serious part of your health regimen. Add humor in other ways: books, movies, cat videos, comedy clubs, blogs, or time with a furry friend or a child. Try out an improv class and say "yes, and . . ." more often.

> Talk to your neighbors. Look them in the eye, say hello, and chitchat. Do something unexpectedly kind. A culture of kindness is contagious. Learn enough about them that you can offer to help out when something comes up, or vice versa. Consider a neighborhood potluck, coffee hour, walking group, board game night, tulip bulb planting, or book/clothes swap.

> Having worked in coffee shops, I add this one: say hello and talk to the person who hands you your drink. If you are a

regular, learn her name. Ask her how her day is going. Every bit of positive connection helps.

> If you are doing an activity anyway, like working out, attending an event, going to the store or library, etc., see if you can do it with a friend. It becomes bonus social time. Even if they decline, the invite alone is a nice way to connect.

> Consider adopting a pet. Offer to dog-sit for a friend or accompany her to the dog park. Volunteer at a shelter, or foster a cat or rabbit or guinea pig or a service dog in training. Consider if your four-legged friend might be a good pet therapy volunteer for a local community center or hospital.

> Also, as a wise friend suggested, make a point of spending time alone, too, and getting comfortable in your own skin. It will help you reach out to others.

Chapter Four

Work: What You Do

Love and work are the cornerstones of our humanness.
—DR. SIGMUND FREUD

When I greeted Sylvie, a new patient in the clinic, I thought she was approaching her sixties. While her hair and makeup were neatly done, her once-tailored tweed suit now hung off her thin frame, and her handshake felt noticeably limp. When Sylvie smiled, I noticed her receded gums and that a tooth in back was missing. I flipped open her medical record and had to double-check the name. The chart said Sylvie was forty-eight years old. *Why did she look so run down?*

Sylvie had come in that day for a second opinion on her multiple physical concerns. She'd already had an extensive work-up by another doctor, which had turned up no diagnosis. Something was wrong, but it wasn't going to show up in her bloodwork or imaging report. As we talked, I learned Sylvie had spent her whole career at a major magazine publisher in Manhattan. Right out of high school, she started working in the mailroom. Even though the pay was low, she felt lucky to get in the door of such a glamorous company. Over the years, she'd worked her way up through various roles to executive assistant. She always came in early and often stayed late, putting in demanding ten-hour days despite the long commute. On special projects she often worked weekends too. Her job was her life. And not in a good way.

Morale at the company was low. There'd been multiple leadership changes over the past decade and most of her friends had been laid off. In the sea of new faces, people didn't know or value her years of dedication. She'd had a rotation of hotshot young bosses who were quick to criticize her without warning, and she felt her every move was "micromanaged." Her current boss, Aiden, once called her cell phone shouting and demanding to know where she was. She was on the toilet. Sylvie's back bothered her from the long hours sitting at her computer and she worried about how much pain medicine she required to get through the day. She was also having frequent headaches. Despite not feeling well, she kept adding more to her plate to appease her boss. She left many of her vacation days unused. Sylvie worried her work was taking a major toll on her health.

Sylvie is not unusual. Today many people spend long, stressful hours in the workplace. As we've traveled through the rings of the hidden factors, we've seen that our relationships and social supports influence our health in powerful ways. Now we'll look at another crucial determinant to our well-being: our jobs.

We spend about a third of our lives at work, and that's not including commute time. Despite the long hours, it's estimated that at least half of us are dissatisfied with our jobs.[1] The American Psychological Association reports job pressure, such as feeling overwhelmed or tension with coworkers or a boss, is the top cause of personal stress in the US, even ahead of money and health concerns. Forty percent of Americans report their job is "very or extremely stressful."[2] And 2016 data from the General Social Survey found that half of workers feel "burned out."[3] Burnout is a mix of exhaustion, cynicism, and inefficiency and is considered the reason half of all people leave their workplaces.[4]

Sylvie's burnout was literally written on her face. When we're under stress at work, others may comment on our "haggard" look. After a year on the hospital wards at medical school, I remember a concerned advisor commenting how I looked "aged." (Since he was in his late seventies, I didn't take it too personally.) And we've seen how our presidents can look like they've matured a decade after a four-year term. But can work stress really account for the kind of extreme physiological change I witnessed in Sylvie?

Endocrinologist Dr. Hans Selye was fascinated by this very question. He asked how someone can feel or even look unwell with no diagnosable disease. As an ambitious young researcher, Dr. Selye aimed to make his professional mark by identifying a new hormone. He devised an experiment where he injected lab rats with different toxins and expected different hormonal reactions. Only he kept getting the same biological response no matter what toxin he exposed the rat to. He grew so frustrated and discouraged by his results, he considered quitting science altogether.[5]

When dealing with something that doesn't make sense, there are two main options: ignore it or explore it. As Robert Frost advised, "The best way out is always through."[6] Fortunately, sitting in his lab, Dr. Selye worked through his perplexing results for a "Eureka!" moment that has changed our understanding of biology ever since. His important discovery was hidden in plain sight.

In 1936 Dr. Selye published a breakthrough paper in the journal *Nature* on a health condition he called general adaptation syndrome (GAS).[7] His paper described the general way a body physiologically adapts under a variety of threats. His discovery's more famous stage name is "stress." He'd identified the common stress response.

Negotiating stress successfully is a key component of life. Dr. Selye said, "The only person without stress is a dead person." All living things must navigate adversity to live. The source of stress is almost irrelevant. Whether there is a lion in pursuit, a war on your doorstep, an ice storm pelting your home, or a hostile boss looking over your shoulder—your body perceives it as a life-or-death, fight-or-flight situation. It reacts with a cascade of hormones: a burst of adrenaline and a biological chain reaction. In the short run, the immediate stress response is helpful for staying alive. In the long run, too much unchecked stress causes intense wear and tear on the body—known as an allosteric load—which can take a serious toll on health.

Allostasis is the body's neurohormonal way of maintaining stability in persistent turbulence. However, chronic activation of the body's stress response system—known as the hypothalamic-pituitary-adrenal (HPA) axis—takes a cumulative toll. It can shorten life span if not alleviated. We now understand that pro-inflammatory cytokines released by the stress response give people "sick behaviors" like wanting to crawl into bed, feeling down, and zapping motivation. Resting is helpful in the short term, but if the stress is prolonged—such as with an ongoing threat like an unstable, unsafe, or chronically stressful job—it is in itself an independent risk factor for many diseases such as infection, type 2 diabetes, osteoporosis, heart attack, stroke, cancer, and mental illness.[8] Increased stress also contributes to poor lifestyle choices such as smoking, drinking alcohol, doing drugs, and eating nachos with imitation cheese from that sketchy corner deli.

Work stress isn't something that happens overnight. Usually it's prolonged and involves attacks on multiple fronts. It may take the form of a chronically overwhelming job, boss, coworker—or all three. As with Sylvie, it may be also compounded by a company's financial instability and a threat to one's own position. The result can be dramatic physiological change. That run-down look I noted, which aged her ten years, reflects what's happening inside her body on a cellular level. If she doesn't make a change in her work situation, she may unknowingly shave years off her life. In Sylvie's case, the hidden factor of work may literally be killing her.

On the flip side, there are people in demanding or repetitive jobs who seem to roll with stress well. So what's different about these situations?

Tommy's story offers some clues. Tommy spent his career with New York City's sanitation services. While working as a garbage man at first take may seem like a thankless, dirty job, Tommy loved his work. He told me, "I always liked being outdoors, not cooped up in some office." Plus, he got a kick out of driving the big trucks. Now well into his sixties with salt-and-pepper hair, his childlike joy was obvious as he said, "There's nothin' like being out there on the roads first thing in the morning right after it snows." He took pride in his years of keeping the city looking its best. "Some people say New York is dirty. But we worked hard every day to make it beautiful." It seems some of the happiest, most well-adjusted people don't necessarily have a lot of material wealth or the corner office, but they do feel pride in their work.

There are countless others much like Tommy. Guillermo works as a hospital janitor and brightens up not only the hospital floors and patient rooms, but also the day of everyone he meets. When he is off, the place is noticeably gloomier. Julie works the cash register at a local grocery store. She enjoys talking with her colleagues and customers, calculating exact change quickly in her head, and the contentment of a job well done at the end of the day. Drew always felt an emotional connection with animals. After he got laid off from his bank teller job during the recession, he started walking his neighbors' dogs. He discovered he looks forward to caring for his furry friends far more than any shift he ever worked at the bank. Plus, he's never been in better shape, often clocking well over fifteen thousand steps a day. Jackie, a home health aide, takes pride that she has perfected the art of bathing clients who can't care for themselves, a surprisingly tricky skill.[9] The board of education offered Patty a job as a principal numerous times, but she politely declined every time. She knew that being in the classroom with first-graders brought her far more tangible rewards. While cash in the wallet is nice, a person can be rich with satisfaction in her work.

Dignity at work is crucial. We may spend a lot of time thinking about how to get the best, most perfect job where we save the world and earn a gazillion dollars doing it. But what often gets lost in this daydream is the simple joy found in working. And the difference between Sylvie and Tommy is that daily dignity, autonomy, and respect matter. Especially for our health.

We know this in part because of a series of landmark longitudinal studies starting in the 1960s looking at health outcomes in civil servants in the Whitehall area of London. Similar to the rabbit studies, the research was designed for another purpose entirely: simply to look at physiological risk factors for heart and lung disease. What turned out to be most fascinating about the studies was an accidental finding.

The researchers chose to study civil servants because they were a large group of people who stuck with their jobs over the years. They would be easy to locate for follow-up. Plus, all participants had health care through the national health plan, which controlled for access to medical care. In addition, everyone was employed, with a fairly narrow range of salaries, which helped control for the role of income on health.

The first Whitehall study followed 17,530 male civil servants for ten years, starting in 1967. It measured potential cardiovascular disease risk factors such as high blood pressure, cholesterol, weight, and smoking. As a matter of "housekeeping," researchers also recorded the employment grade the men were in the hierarchical agency. Seven and a half years into the study there was an unmistakable and completely unanticipated finding. The strongest predictor of death from heart disease wasn't cholesterol or blood pressure. It was a man's employment grade. From the boss in the corner office to the man sweeping the floor, there was a clear gradient. (A health gradient is another causal clue that makes an epidemiologist fall off her chair.)

Sir Michael Marmot was a researcher on the study, and he initially couldn't make sense of the results.[10] In the 1970s, there was an assumption that those with the

> The strongest predictor of death from heart disease wasn't cholesterol or blood pressure. It was a man's employment grade.

most responsibility at work had the most stressful jobs, and thus would have the highest risk of heart attack. But the data showed exactly the opposite. It wasn't the boss in the corner office dropping dead. Instead, people at the lowest grades died from heart disease at three to six times the rate as those at the highest grade. And the striking inverse association between rank and coronary heart disease occurred in a stepwise gradient along employment grade. In other words, the top administrators had less heart disease than the professionals (such as doctors and lawyers), and the professionals had less than the clerical staff, and the clerical staff had less than lower support staff, such as the maintenance crew. The higher one's status in the organization, the better the odds of a healthy heart.[11]

Consistent with other studies, those at the lowest ranks were more overweight and more likely to smoke and have higher blood pressure. They were also curiously shorter in height, perhaps suggestive of childhood nutritional differences. While these known risk factors for mortality likely contributed to an early demise, the employment grade finding still held even after researchers controlled for all these differences. A person whose job was lower in the hierarchy had a higher risk of death. Period. And it wasn't just from heart disease. It was from all causes.

To confirm the results and expand on the findings, researchers repeated the study with a new group of 10,314 civil servants starting in 1985. This time, they included women. The Whitehall II study, which was published in 1991 in *The Lancet*, confirmed the social gradient between status and health found in the first Whitehall study.[12] In addition, this time they asked careful questions to try to understand the participants' experience on the job. They asked subjects how much in control they felt of their day, how fairly coworkers treated them, how valued they were, and how satisfying they found the work.[13] Researchers also asked the subjects how healthy they felt. One particularly curious finding of the Whitehall II study was how those with lower employment status both had more symptoms *and* felt more pessimistic about their health.

While the Whitehall studies originally looked for biological risk factors for heart disease, what they uncovered was an unexpected link between the mind and the body. The researchers found that when people felt socially supported by their supervisors, could make their own decisions during the day, felt rewarded and valued for their efforts on the job, and were engaged by their work, their mental and physical health benefited.[14] In addition, those who felt socially supported in a positive work environment took less sick leave and company healthcare expenses were 50 percent less.[15]

> When people felt socially supported by their supervisors, could make their own decisions during the day, felt rewarded and valued for their efforts on the job, and were engaged by their work, their mental and physical health benefited.

Most people would say having a good doctor is important to health, but this data implies that having a good manager is also critical for avoiding disease. Managers who support and value their employees, who trust them and value their autonomy, and who promote the dignity of work help both humans and organizations thrive.[16] When you don't feel under threat or scrutiny, you have more available working memory to problem solve and be creative. Indeed, a study of nineteen thousand people published in the *Harvard Business Review* found that those who feel treated with dignity at work are far more (55 percent more) engaged.[17] In addition, an economics study looking at millions of responses from Gallup daily polls over the years found workers who feel they have a supervisor who is a "partner" versus a "boss" are significantly happier. The difference for those with a partner boss was equivalent to a doubling of household income.[18] If you are a manager, know you play a lead role in the health of your staff. And their well-being and happiness will help drive your success.

So let's say you feel stressed out at work and you don't have a great boss or you face other constraints like low pay or high physical and emotional demands. What can you do besides quitting your job, to allow yourself to feel more in control, gain more resilience, and craft more dignity?

One first step is to find your flow. Since I was a teenager, I've held many jobs, from folding dress shirts at an outlet mall to tallying pesticide use by California farmers. One of my happiest was working as a barista at a coffee shop in Lake Tahoe, California. Even though I made just enough money to live on that summer, I found the work highly satisfying. I enjoyed getting to know the customers and got immersed in the art of trying to make the perfect cappuccino. I lost track of time in the rhythm of the espresso machine: the tamping of the handles, the *woosh* of frothing milk, and the wiggle of the pour. That intense concentration while working on a skill is what psychologist Mihaly Csikszentmihalyi calls flow. This playful state of mental absorption in a task is associated with reduced stress, increased happiness, health promotion, and longevity.[19] Finding flow brings joy and positive experience to whatever task you do.[20]

The joy of flow might relate to what former Harvard professor and spiritual teacher Ram Dass posed in the 1970s: "Be here now." Meanwhile, studies show that we are not mentally present in what we are physically doing nearly half the time. Our minds love to visit the past, dream of the future, and think about what's for dinner, yet studies show that we are happiest when we're living in the moment. And research shows less mind wandering is far more predictive of one's happiness in salary. Even if the activity in the present is unpleasant, like commuting, people report feeling far happier when focused on the task at hand rather than letting their mind drift. Studies where people are asked multiple times a day about their mood through a smartphone app show that mind wandering precedes unhappiness, rather than the other way around.[21]

In addition to finding flow, the ability to brush things off, feel up to a challenge, or take a break helps reduce the risk of disease. For example, one large study found that people who took renewal breaks (like a short walk) at work reported they were 50 percent more engaged in their jobs and felt twice as healthy as those who were not encouraged to take such breaks.[22] In a profound example of this, a study of over twenty-three thousand Greek adults published in *JAMA Archives* found people who nap regularly are less likely to die from heart disease than those who don't.

People who nap regularly are less likely to die from heart disease than those who don't.

For working men, a midday siesta reduced the risk of death from heart disease 64 percent.[23] Perhaps that's part of why Spain, with its culturally sanctioned nap time, is expected to overtake Japan as the world's longest-living country in 2040.[24]

Just like you wouldn't skip your heart medicine, the cardioprotective effects of a brief five- to twenty-minute midday nap suggest you shouldn't skip your nap to power through work, either. While this doesn't mean you should spend the day in bed, it might be a good reason to consider nap pods at the office. I'm reminded of a family friend in his fifties who, on a Monday morning at his stressful finance job, dropped dead from a heart attack. Evidence shows more people have heart attacks and strokes on Mondays, presumably because of the return to work.[25] Could a work culture of regular fifteen-minute power naps have helped him? I wish he'd had that option. Sometimes a break, whether it is a nap, a walk around the block, coffee with a coworker, or a vacation, can change our outlook for the positive.

Part of what makes work both fun and stressful is our relationship with colleagues. Building community at work can go a long way to fostering a feeling that you're supported as a person. Colleagues who ask each other about their weekends on Monday morning or who create space and time during the work week to check in or hang out and do something not work-related are more likely to engage with and feel valued by each other. Workplaces increasingly understand the importance of breaks and community. Twenty-minute guided meditations after lunch and thirty-minute walking groups (see the American Heart Association's Workplace Walking Kit) are on the rise.[26] Engaging coworkers in fun activities they like helps boost team creativity and inclusiveness, as long as everyone remains respectful of family and outside commitments.

No matter what we do to boost community at work, there may still be some team members you'd rather not spend a single minute more with than necessary. Learning to navigate interpersonal conflict is a part of every job. We've all experienced the discomfort of a caustic coworker or workplace bully. I still remember standing there feeling helpless as I watched a senior male doctor publicly berate a nurse (for something minor) to the point of tears. Whether you are witness to it or receiving the tirade yourself, self-care is most important to preserve your well-being, help manage your reaction, and boost your assertiveness. It will also help you act like a pillar for others who may need support.

To increase empathy, recognize his bad behavior usually comes from a place of hurt or pain. As the saying goes, "Hurt people hurt people." Try to put yourself in his shoes to see how out of control he feels. He may not even know the pain he is inflicting. If you can, when emotions are cool, get to know him as a human being. Does he have any pets or kids? What hobbies does he enjoy? Where did he grow up? It's harder to dislike someone when you know him. Plus, the human connection will help you work with him to problem solve and address the unhelpful behavior. If the bullying is harassment, please talk to human resources. You are probably not alone, and your voice may give courage to others to come forward.

Maybe you like your coworkers well enough, but still don't love your job. Then what? One thing you can do is a personal needs assessment. Keep notes for several weeks of what you find fun or meaningful at work. Look for patterns and periods of "flow." This is what Bill Burnett and

Dave Evans, who run Stanford University's Life Design Lab, call a "Good Time Journal."[27] The idea is that once you see what you like, you can focus your time more on what you enjoy and alleviate the less enjoyable parts. Can you plan and pilot some changes to then further tweak your plans going forward? This method of continual improvement is sometimes called a Plan-Do-Study-Act (PDSA) or Deming cycle.

Consider engaging a supervisor or professional coach to help redesign your daily focus and move your career in a direction you want. If you are a manager, mentor your supervisees or partner with someone who can. Consider forming a career support group with people from other fields to give you perspective on your own. Or start a peer mentoring group with your coworkers, which is a model that progressive businesses are using to engage talent and better the business. It usually involves four to eight people at the same level, usually from different departments. Activities may include discussing relevant articles, doing trainings (like conflict resolution or time management or negotiation skills), meeting with leaders and guest speakers, talking about organizational culture, reviewing promotion strategies, and doing some personal goal setting. It is a fun way to network and improve support at work.

Sometimes a stressful situation requires recognizing that we are stronger and more capable than we realize. Like Sylvie, I've found myself stuck in a less-than-desirable work environment where changing my boss or workplace was not an option. As a medical intern, I found a patient pamphlet in a waiting room called "Managing Stress at Work." The red brochure cover showed a cartoon version of an exasperated man with steam and sweat radiating from his head. I saw myself.

While I'm passionate about the field of medicine, the unpredictability of twenty-four-hour overnight call, with constantly interrupted sleep, dying patients, and little downtime, wore on me. There was one understaffed city hospital I covered regularly where the pager went off so incessantly throughout the night that sometimes I could not physically return all the pages. I was always terrified that I had missed something. The beeps would range from a stool softener order to Mr. Acktar having chest pain. If things got really bad, they'd page me over the PA system too. I always needed to be in three places at once. My blood pressure crept up enough that year that my doctor recommended starting a hypertension agent.

I slipped the pamphlet into my white coat pocket to read privately. The only problem was, even looking at it, I felt my blood pressure rise. Intellectually knowing stress is bad for health doesn't stop stress. The problem is that stress is braided into the fabric of our daily lives—no matter how much we try to avoid it, there it is. And if none of the usual strategies are working to combat that stress, sometimes more dramatic change is required.

When I started in academic medicine, a beloved mentor took me for coffee and spoke confidentially. At the time, I did not know it, but she had dedicated herself to career advancement at a tremendous personal cost to her own health. As a parting word, she told me, "Work hard, but remember, institutions don't love you back." I took her words to mean, "Don't sacrifice everything else that's important to you for career advancement alone." As comedian Amy Poehler put it, "Treat your career like a bad boyfriend."[28] In other words, it's good to invest in your passions, but jobs come and go. It's also a reminder that you're not married to your work: you could leave.

So how do we know when it is time to leave a job? The red flags include feeling chronically unsupported, undervalued, threatened, or like your dignity has corroded. Just like in a relationship, where you draw the line will vary by individual circumstance. But please take your mental well-being and the dignity you are accorded daily seriously. Some jobs can get downright abusive, and the mental and physical costs far outweigh the benefits. If you can't make it work, realize that leaving is a form of self-respect too. There are steps we can take to make the most of a less-than-ideal situation, but sometimes for your own good you do have to make a plan, pack a bag, call your sister, and move on.

Before making a big career choice, I'd like to raise an important consideration. It's along the lines of not marrying for money. Many of us associate better jobs with a higher salary and a higher salary with more happiness. But what we know from watching all those reality TV shows is backed up by research: the relationship between money and happiness is messy. A study in the 1980s found that receiving $5,000 was the equivalent of only a 2 percent boost in happiness. Meanwhile, each happy friend is the equivalent of being given $20,000.[29] Friendship really is more precious than gold. Perhaps a job with more flexibility to spend time with loved ones is a better bonus than stock options.

Money is helpful to well-being, but only to a point. Some money in our pockets does contribute to improved health.[30] In the US, the poorest households (making less than $22,500) had three times the rate of health problems than those making more than $47,700 per year. In addition, those in the bottom third of incomes skipped needed medical care one out of five times as compared to one out of twenty-five in the top third of incomes.[31] As Charles Dickens's work illustrates, poverty exacerbates misfortune.

But, as we will discuss in chapter 10, happiness does not rise continually with income either.[32] A 2018 study published in *Nature* looking at 1.7 million people worldwide in 164 countries found incomes beyond $60,000 to $75,000 (in US dollars) didn't add much to emotional well-being. This is consistent with other research done at Princeton University by economists Daniel Kahneman and Angus Deaton in 2010. They also found that well-being, defined as "the frequency and intensity of experiences of joy, stress, sadness, anger, and affection that make one's life pleasant or unpleasant," levels out after about $75,000.[33] After basic needs are met, more money may bring some bonus life satisfaction, but it doesn't bring more day-to-day happiness.

Happiness does not rise continually with income.

In fact, our rat race with more money as the reward may inadvertently create more misery for most of us. British epidemiologist Richard Wilkinson studies how social inequality and wide income gaps erode social cohesion, population well-being, and health outcomes. Using data from the World Bank and the United Nations, his work demonstrates that wide income gaps between the wealthiest and the poorest in a country strongly correlate with worse health outcomes across a variety of standard measures such as life expectancy, infant mortality, homicides, imprisonment, teen pregnancies, obesity, mental illness, and substance use. Even the wealthy people in a country fare worse than expected when there's a wide national income gap. As you may recall, out of the thirty-two most affluent countries in the world, the US ranked worst on the wealth-health gap.[34] There is reason to believe this is only going to worsen, since 1 percent of the world's population has increasingly more wealth than the other 99 percent combined.[35]

Many of us live life feeling, "I'll just be happy once I achieve some goal or make a certain amount of money," only to discover once the goal arrives or the cash hits the bank that happiness was not included. While the idea that money can't buy us love isn't a new one, sometimes it takes a personal tragedy to truly understand the message. Google X's chief business officer Mo Gawdat felt a deep sense of dissatisfaction and suffering, despite having two Rolls-Royces in the garage. After the sudden death of his twenty-one-year-old son, Ali, from a medical error in a routine procedure, the equation of Mo's life changed overnight.

Since Ali's death, Gawdat has dedicated himself to what he calls a "moonshot for humanity" to reduce greed, ego, and showing off. His goal is to have one billion people commit to making happiness—not material wealth—their top priority.[36] He believes if we each refocus on human flourishing and talk to at least two people about our actions, we could build a kinder nation and world, with direct impact on our workplaces. Contrary to popular belief, studies show that happiness brings success, not the other way around. For instance, one review of 250 studies found that positive affect—the hallmark of well-being—precedes success in domains such as income, work performance, and health.[37]

Working impacts our health far beyond the cash we make and our access to medical care.[38] The evidence shows we need to reframe job success from paychecks and benefits to dignity and positive engagement. As we saw with Sylvie, the respect we accord each other in and out of the workplace matters deeply for our health. Emotional well-being, including happiness, is far more valuable than more money or prestige. Work at its best, no matter what the job, can infuse our lives with a sense of contentment and satisfaction that contributes to our wellness. As we'll discuss in the next chapter, sometimes we can learn to align what we do with who we are and our greater sense of purpose.

EXPAND YOUR TOOL KIT
Work

Given how much time we spend at work and the impact our jobs have on our health, it's useful to think about ways we might make it more enjoyable for ourselves. Here are some ideas to consider in your process of self-discovery.

› Develop your own outlets outside of work. Time with friends, family, pets, sports leagues, support groups, or hobbies puts stressful interactions at work in perspective and allows you to recharge.

› Can you reframe some work stress as a challenge? Be aware of bodily sensations of anxiety and see if you can reframe it as "excitement." (As one of my favorite children's authors, Cooper Edens, says, "If you have butterflies in your stomach, invite them into your heart.")

› Make sure your energy is spent on the important tasks. Clarify what is critical to your boss or manager. Be clear on requirements and expectations. If you feel stretched, ask her what to deprioritize so you can get the essential tasks done well.

› People-pleasing and always saying yes to everything risks burnout, big time. To reduce this risk, start by setting boundaries, which may include telling coworkers that evenings or weekends are reserved for family or personal time. Don't read (or send) work emails outside of business hours. This takes the pressure off everyone else too. Also, pause before you accept new projects. Will it interfere with time needed for your current priority or cut into personal time? What is the trade-off? Recognize that time is your most valuable currency.

▸ Consider appointing a chief happiness officer (it may sound a little too cheerful, but hey, it works at Google). If one doesn't exist, appoint yourself. Find ambassadors. Consider the Science of Happiness at Work Professional Certificate program from UC Berkeley's Greater Good Science Center.[39]

▸ Find a way to offer people kudos for a job well done. For example, one San Diego law office collects stories of teamwork, creativity, and going the extra mile each month and then shares them aloud at a lunchtime celebration. They give prizes (i.e., coffee gift cards) for recipients. UnitedHealthcare rewards staff for not only doing good work but pointing out the good work of colleagues. There are lots of creative ways to draw attention to good work, boost morale, and create a positive work culture.

▸ Make a personal policy of not talking behind coworkers' backs. It erodes a supportive culture. Politely excuse yourself when others engage in this behavior or let them know that that hasn't been your experience. This doesn't mean tolerating bad behaviors, but instead finding a way to offer more direct feedback and encourage others to do the same.

▸ Can you close the conference room door and meditate for ten minutes or take a nap during the day? If you don't telecommute, does your office have nap pods? If you're the boss, set a good self-care example and use them.

▸ Please take vacation and the occasional mental health day to reboot. Research shows this boosts creativity and reduces sick days overall. Plus it makes you a more pleasant coworker, seriously.

➤ Check out Mo Gawdat's happiness library at onebillionhappy .org and Bill Burnett and Dave Evans's Designing Your Life website (https://designingyour.life) to get ideas on how to reframe your work and life to boost your joy.

➤ Pay attention to the culture in your workplace. If it's not one where you feel supported and encouraged, you can try to tweak it or move on. While change is stressful, it can also be invigorating.

Chapter Five

Education:
Learning Your Purpose

*Your purpose in life is to find your purpose and
give your whole heart and soul to it.*
—BUDDHA

At Dr. Carola Eisenberg's hundredth birthday party, seating for all the guests was a problem. Her son Dr. Larry Guttmacher, my longtime mentor, joked that they needed a larger venue. The Argentinean restaurant, complete with tango dancers, wasn't big enough for all the colleagues and friends from Dr. Eisenberg's life whom she wanted to invite. Almost two months later, my son Ryan, then eight, and I visited Dr. Eisenberg's lovely home in Cambridge for dinner. Ryan, who shares a birthday with Dr. Eisenberg, ninety-two years apart, brought her a Wonder Woman figurine as a present. It was a fitting tribute. Not only had Dr. Eisenberg made it to one hundred years old, her impressive career would inspire anyone. How had one person managed to accomplish so much?

Dr. Eisenberg's parents had encouraged her education from an early age and sparked her innate curiosity about the human condition. Despite humble beginnings, she studied social work and then became one of the few women to attend medical school in her native Argentina in the 1940s. After graduation, she accepted an offer in the US to train as a child psychiatrist at the Johns Hopkins Hospital in Baltimore. When her first husband (Larry's father) died unexpectedly from leukemia, she made her way to Boston. There she became the first female dean of students at the Massachusetts Institute of Technology and then at Harvard Medical School.

The night we visited her at her home, the doorman asked if we would mind giving Dr. Eisenberg a book that a friend had left for her. It was heavy, with a complicated academic title, written in tiny print. Dr. Eisenberg seemed delighted to receive the scholarly tome, and I have no doubt she planned to plunge into it later. Her elegant apartment displayed a similar spirit of inquiry: artwork from adventures around the world, plants, and photos. After Ryan and I arrived, Dr. Eisenberg said in her lovely Argentinean accent, "Before I tell you more about me, I want to hear more about you." Her curiosity knew no bounds. Where did I grow up? What was my family like? Did I have siblings? When Ryan made himself comfortable with a book, stretched across the back of her couch like a cat, Dr. Eisenberg laughed. She said with a warm smile, "I love it!" Ryan grinned and then got lost in his book.

In Dr. Eisenberg's retirement, she helped form Physicians for Human Rights. Having seen the negative effects of civil unrest on well-being in her homeland, she spent much of her career thinking about the hidden factors of health. The group, whose slogan is "Through evidence, change is possible," shared the 1997 Nobel Peace Prize for their work on reducing land mines globally. The group has several missions, including helping unjustly imprisoned medical workers around the world. Not the typical encore career. From our conversation, it was clear that Dr. Eisenberg still participates in groups relating to health-care improvement and human rights. When it became too much for her to travel in the harsh Boston winter to a favorite organization's headquarters for meetings, her colleagues came to her house instead.

Dr. Eisenberg's rich social life seems a natural extension of all her different intellectual pursuits. She stays in touch with scores of former students, saying warmly, "They come by and want to tell me about their accomplishments. I just love to see them and their families." She often hosts potlucks for former colleagues, students, and friends. I asked her how often she has visitors, and she said on average four to five times a week.

As we've seen, the hidden factors of Dr. Eisenberg's impressive one-on-one connections, social supports, and healthy work environment undoubtedly contributed to her longevity. But as we said our goodbyes that evening, I was struck anew by the sheer exuberance and vigor of her unusual life. From my public health training, I knew education was a hidden factor in health, and surely Dr. Eisenberg's lifelong love of learning had something to do with her stamina and remarkable achievements. But something else seemed to be contributing to Dr. Eisenberg's vitality. I had traveled to Cambridge looking for answers and left with a question: *How can we all live such a full life?*

Believe it or not, the answer may lurk in pond scum.

As a graduate student at Yale in the mid-1970s, Australian-born scientist Dr. Elizabeth Blackburn, the same illustrious scientist responsible for reuniting me and Dr. Arthur Barsky, studied the one-celled organism *Tetrahymena thermophila*, aka pond scum. These organisms are useful to researchers because they have ample short linear chromosomes. Examining the cells, she identified a short simple sequence of base pairs (TTGGGG) at the end of their DNA, which sometimes repeated fifty times over. Curiously, the repeats varied in length from organism to organism.[1] Dr. Blackburn then asked a question that would eventually earn her a Nobel Prize and change the way we think about aging forever: "How did the repeats get there?"[2]

The DNA buffers, known as telomeres, are essential for chromosome stability—the genetic equivalent of the plastic tips on shoelaces that protect the lace from fraying. The tips were first noticed by researchers Hermann Müller and Barbara McClintock in the 1930s, even before scientists learned that DNA carried genetic information. Dr. Blackburn noticed that every time a cell divided, the cell's telomeres got a bit shorter. Cells can only divide so many times in their life span. When the telomeres become too short, the cell dies. This led Dr. Blackburn and her colleagues to wonder if the opposite were also true. Perhaps if telomeres could stay long in healthy cells, death wouldn't be inevitable. After all, some animals' telomeres rejuvenate. Certain kinds of tortoises, lobsters, and jellyfish enjoy immortality unless they become ill, injured, or captured.[3]

For humans, the longer our telomeres, the longer our lives and the healthier we are. Shorter telomeres predict a shorter life and increase the risk of death from a variety of diseases such as heart disease, infection, cancer, and dementia. When people of the same age are divided into two groups based on telomere length, the half with longer telomeres live an average of five years longer than those with shorter telomeres.[4]

Eventually, Dr. Blackburn figured out the answer to her question. In 2009 she and two colleagues, Dr. Carol Greider and Dr. Jack Szostak, won the Nobel Prize in Medicine for the discovery of the enzyme telomerase, which rebuilds shortened telomeres by adding back lost bits of nucleotides. Increased activity of telomerase slows telomere shortening and elongates telomeres. Now, *what* increases that activity is the fascinating part that we will explore together. While cancer cells hijack this process and greedily flip on telomerase only for themselves, regulation of telomerase activity has huge implications for aging. Notably, the research indicated that whether our telomeres rejuvenate or shorten isn't determined simply by our genes.

If people's telomerase is genetically determined, then it would follow that identical twins, barring any serious accident, would have telomeres about the same length and would likely die around the same time. But that's not true. Swedish researchers looked at the telomeres of older identical twins. They found that the twin with shorter telomeres was three times likelier to die first.[5] Another study from Spain found that identical twins are genetically indistinguishable at birth; however, as they age, they start to show remarkable differences mediated through epigenetic changes. These differences were nearly all located in the telomere regions. The less of their lives the twins spent together, the greater the differences.[6] The twin studies seem to confirm that the lives we lead have an important impact on telomerase activity—and, hence, on aging.

Living a life filled with prolonged stress negatively affects our telomere length and our health. Like Sylvie, the executive assistant whose job took a toll, prolonged stress also affects our appearance. Individuals with shorter telomeres look more haggard. It turns out, appearance is a fair proxy for telomere length. If two genetically identical rats have different telomere lengths, the one with shorter telomeres will look more ragtag. Truncated telomeres are associated with skin aging, poor wound healing, and graying hair.[7] Interestingly, the Guinness Record holder for oldest living fish, Tish (whom I'll discuss in the next chapter), changed color from brilliant orange to off-white in his later years. His golden years were not so golden.

It seems the relationship between life stress, telomeres, and disease provides a mechanism for the hidden connection between the mind and the cell, our social world, and our health. Thus it follows that reducing stress increases telomerase activity in healthy cells and decreases the risk of disease. And indeed, a growing body of research suggests that lifestyle changes—such as exercise, deep relaxation (meditation, yoga), healthy diet (more plant-based), and increased social ties (hanging out with supportive friends and colleagues)—may protect or increase telomere lengths.

Dr. Dean Ornish, along with Dr. Blackburn and Dr. Elissa Epel, published a series of studies in *The Lancet* that found a dose-response (or proportional relationship) between degree of lifestyle change and improvement in a variety of health factors, including telomerase activity. The researchers followed a group of men diagnosed with prostate cancer who made a lifestyle change, adopting healthy habits, such as diet, physical activity, stress management, and social support. At a five-year follow-up, the results showed a significant increase in telomeres from the start of the study. The longer someone stayed on the program, the longer his telomeres. The control group didn't make lifestyle changes and had shorter telomeres by the end of the study.[8]

And here again is that incredible link between the mind and the cell. It seems mental well-being and optimism correlate with longer telomeres and longer survival.[9] In particular, a study done at Yale University showed that middle-aged and older adults who had a positive attitude about aging lived 7.6 years longer than those who did not. That is the same benefit as maintaining normal blood pressure, exercising regularly, and not smoking.[10] Maybe a serious part of a good health regimen is watching stereotype shattering shows about aging, like *The Golden Girls*.

Perhaps Dr. Eisenberg was born with naturally long telomeres. Or maybe her remarkable life—a life filled to the brim with meaningful intellectual pursuits and related social connection—helped keep her telomerase active, contributing to her health and longevity. Maybe her social and intellectual activities buffered her against significant stressors such as political turmoil in her homeland and being twice widowed. But another factor may also be at work. As the research suggests, factors that increase our telomerase activity, including a positive outlook, increase our life span. And part of what stands out about Dr. Eisenberg—and Dr. Blackburn too—is her sense of optimism, meaning, and drive. Which led me to ask, *Is a life full of purpose, often connected to a lifelong love of learning, another hidden factor in health?*

The evidence shows a sense of purpose, and being engaged in your day-to-day is indeed health protective. A significant decrease in stress and inflammatory markers is noted in people with high *eudaimonic well-being*, a term that describes striving for a noble, meaningful purpose. A focus on meaning and self-realization not only lowers daily salivary cortisol levels and pro-inflammatory markers but offers some impressive health advantages.[11] A meta-analysis combining ten prospective studies found that a high sense of purpose in life or usefulness (or, as they say in Okinawa, *ikigai*) is associated with a significantly reduced risk of all causes of death.[12] People who infuse purpose into their day-to-day sleep better, are less susceptible to viruses, and have healthier hearts. Higher purpose is associated with a reduced need for coronary artery bypass surgery (CABG) and cardiac stenting procedures. Other benefits range from a lower risk of stroke (72 percent lower risk) and heart disease (44 percent lower risk) to better outcomes when they are sick, such as with reduced cancer spread, spinal cord injuries, multiple sclerosis, autoimmune disorders, or dementia.[13]

> People who infuse purpose into their day-to-day sleep better, are less susceptible to viruses, and have healthier hearts.

Feeling connected to purpose and passion is particularly important for cognitive functioning as the brain ages. A study published in *JAMA*'s

Archives series followed nine hundred older adults living in the Chicago area for up to eight years. They found that people who reported a high feeling of life purpose had nearly a two and a half times reduced risk of developing Alzheimer's disease versus those who reported a low feeling of life purpose. In addition, the people who reported a greater sense of purpose staved off cognitive impairment better as the years rolled on. The greater the sense of life purpose, the greater the benefit. This did not vary among demographics and persisted after researchers controlled for social network size, medical conditions, and even depression. (After all, purpose and happiness are not exactly the same thing.)[14]

In a related study, people who reported a greater sense of purpose had better cognitive functioning even with advancing Alzheimer's disease. Even if a person's brain on autopsy showed lots of disease, such as numerous plaques and tangles, a high sense of purpose in life helped them function better.[15] Finding meaning in daily events, pursuing goal-directed behavior, and feeling relevant have a powerful neuroprotective effect. This reminds me of the most prolific and arguably inspiring mathematician of all time, Paul Erdős. He lived his life fully with the unique

> People who reported a greater sense of purpose had better cognitive functioning even with advancing Alzheimer's disease.

singular focus on solving equations with his mathematician friends. He would reportedly show up on their doorstep to stay with them and announce, "My brain is open!"[16] In his lifetime, he published over 1,500 papers with 507 coauthors, to the point that the collaborative distance between him and another mathematician is known as the "Erdős number." He died as he wished at age eighty-three: at a conference in Warsaw just hours after solving a pesky geometry problem.[17]

I think back to my dinner with Dr. Eisenberg, who seemed so passionate about helping others and found purpose in her ongoing work and the ability to make life choices in pursuit of that purpose. I also think about Dr. Blackburn, who, in her late sixties, has a youthful exuberance and seems deeply driven to solve the riddle of telomeres. I once moderated a talk for Dr. Blackburn at an enormous convention hall in San

Francisco. I felt like the opening act for the Beatles. Her rock-star status is well deserved and stems from her clear focus and passion. There must be a way we can all increase our odds of being as fortunate as these two remarkable women.

There is one clear path to developing a sense of meaning and purpose in our lives. Remember that book the doorman gave me to give to Dr. Eisenberg? Not to mention her great interest in understanding the lives of the people around her. Both provide a clue to yet another hidden factor to health, one continuously underestimated yet perhaps the mother of all hidden factors. It's one with which you're already familiar, since you've been curious enough to pick up this book.

It's learning. Simply learning.

Starting in the 1970s, researchers noticed a relationship between education and health measures such as infectious diseases, smoking, alcohol use, diabetes, obesity, and heart disease.[18] For example, a patient without a high school diploma is at double the risk for diabetes as a college graduate (15 percent versus 7 percent) and three times more likely to die from the disease if he didn't graduate high school than if he had taken some college courses.[19] A woman with a college degree is significantly less likely to be obese than a woman without (25 percent versus 40 percent).[20] A large study of 27,033 white men and women in Chicago found a statistically significant inverse association between number of years spent in school and blood pressure.[21] In addition, compelling evidence shows that education protects against telomere shortening, particularly for people of color regardless of income.[22] Doctors often ask about risk factors such as sugar, calorie, or salt intake, but what about information intake?

Increasing evidence shows that the health-protective effects of education are dramatic. Low education, meaning less than a high school diploma, carries the same health risk as smoking.[23] Joey is in his thirties, has a high school diploma, and works a minimum-wage position. Rather than resembling the health of his peers who went off to college, Joey's health profile is closer to that of a sixty-year-old who attended some college. Evidence even suggests that having a child graduate college extends parents' lives by several years.[24] So maybe the homework battles are worth the trouble after all.

Education appears protective of health both in terms of years lived and quality of life. As with the Whitehall studies discussed in chapter 4, there is a clear dose-response (or proportional) gradient between years of school and better health. In the US, people without a high school diploma, especially white women, have been living sicker, shorter lives since the 1990s.[25] Meanwhile, studies suggest that graduating from high school and getting a college degree adds about nine years to someone's life span.[26] Getting a professional degree adds bonus years.[27] And aside from high school and higher education, lifelong learning can add years to our lives.

Studies suggest that graduating from high school and getting a college degree adds about nine years to someone's life span.

And in an incredible study published in the *American Journal of Public Health*, researcher Dr. Steven Woolf and his team examined data on preventable deaths in the US between 1996 and 2002 and found that for every one life saved by biomedicine, education saved eight.[28] According to their data, better education would have saved nearly 1.4 million lives during that time period than the nearly 180,000 lives saved by new drugs and devices alone. That is more people than the entire population of San Francisco whose lives could have been spared by books. It appears the pen is far mightier than the prescription pad.

For every one life biomedicine saves, education saves eight.

As a doctor, I never imagined how much education impacts the health of my patients. This was never covered in medical school or residency. But it makes sense now why so many patients who struggle the most with illness have the lowest education levels. I cried the night I saw Dolores, an incredibly kind woman in her sixties with a gentle manner and a sweet smile. Before she was changed into her hospital gown, I noticed her sunny yellow "Hakuna Matata" T-shirt from Disney's *The Lion King*. She worked for years as a helper at a neighborhood day care and did not have health insurance. Dolores showed up at the emergency room with unbearable abdominal pain that turned out to be advanced cervical cancer—tragically, a preventable disease. After the cause of the pain was discovered and we spoke about her diagnosis, I realized she looked confused beyond just the shock of the news. Eventually, she told me she had only a fourth-grade education.

It appears education provides both direct and indirect benefits to health. Part of education's health boost is a practical component such as how well a patient understands her illness and can read her prescriptions. But educational fulfillment also correlates with better-paying jobs with sick days to go to the doctor, preventive care, and money to fill prescriptions. More education may mean higher earnings to live in a less stressful neighborhood with more access to healthy foods. In addition, education teaches intangibles, such as independent problem solving, grit, and the courage to question the answers.

While most of the health studies just account for quantity of education, such as the number of years in school, quality is important too. When discussing what makes a "good" education, New York City elementary school principal Elena Jaime points out, "There are infinite ways to add up to the number ten." Maybe the purpose of an education isn't to teach us how to think, but to open our eyes to possibilities. And it seems providing opportunities to develop curiosity early, starting with preschool, can equalize other known health factors, such as family income.[29] No matter what form education takes, from Montessori to charter schools, it has the potential to help us increase self-confidence, discover joy in learning, develop social networks, and find fulfillment in navigating and contributing to our world. A good education involves both mind and heart.

Which brings us back to that elusive link between education and purpose, a link that may provide the answer to the question of the "full life" I sought when I left Dr. Eisenberg's. There is an expression that likely originated with Plutarch, "Education is not the filling of a pail, but the lighting of a fire." While the data shows that education in itself is good for health, the best education (formal or informal) goes beyond imparting knowledge to spark the imagination. After all, studies show that emotional health at age sixteen, more than grades, is the best predictor of adult life satisfaction. And a major contributor to emotional health at age sixteen is a child's secondary and elementary school experience.[30] At its best, education challenges the learner to grow as a person, to ask important questions, and to collaborate meaningfully in society. It goes beyond facts or skills alone to focus on intention, fulfillment, and purpose. The best education helps you figure out why something is worth doing at all.

Remember Dr. Nerem from the rabbit studies? In his mid-seventies, after an accomplished research career, Dr. Nerem worked with community partners to develop a program called Project ENGAGES to introduce kids from low-income neighborhoods in Atlanta, Georgia, to STEM (science, technology, engineering, and mathematics) professions. His work at the lab bench led him to the unlikely discovery that attention to social factors—like education—makes for greater innovation in the basic sciences.

Project ENGAGES, short for Engaging New Generations at Georgia Tech through Engineering & Science, connects motivated students with opportunities far beyond the walls of their economically disadvantaged high schools.[31] For the students selected for the program, it is a serious time commitment. The partnering high schools have agreed to adjust the rising juniors' schedules so they can spend mornings in class and afternoons in a lab. Over the school year, they learn research skills, SAT prep, time management, and conflict resolution.

I asked Dr. Nerem, "Why conflict resolution?" He noted that during the application process, the team asks students questions about their lives, such as "Who's your hero?" and "What challenges have you faced?" The teens' answers are eye-opening about the level of adversity they have experienced. He said, "The stories that come out are inspiring . . . and make you wonder about this world." Perhaps telling their stories of adversity is another way that education benefits the students: they find a framework for moving beyond conflict by describing it.

Over 95 percent of Project ENGAGES students go on to college, such as the University of Pennsylvania, Stanford, and Johns Hopkins. Most continue to pursue STEM fields. You could even say those students who engaged with Project ENGAGES and found their imaginations sparked by science have found their life's purpose. And Dr. Nerem did too. I could hear the pride in his voice as, looking back on his many accomplishments in his career, he said "there is nothing more satisfying" than making a difference for the students in Project ENGAGES.

And here's the best part.

Our pursuit of purpose and meaning, like our learning, is a lifelong journey. For example, Nola Ochs was the world's oldest college graduate at age ninety-five. She collected her diploma at Fort Hays State University in Kansas alongside her twenty-one-year-old granddaughter, Alexandra. After graduation they went on a cruise, where Ms. Ochs was a guest lecturer, her lifelong dream. In a video encouraging others to chase their passions she says, "Set a date to begin. Do something. Don't just sit there."[32] Ms. Ochs next pursued her master's degree in liberal studies, which she earned at the age of ninety-eight. She died at the age of 105, just over nine years from when she got her college degree.

Finding our sense of purpose over our lifetime is up to us. Not all of us will have the good fortune and long life of Dr. Eisenberg. Or the intense focus of Dr. Blackburn or Paul Erdős. Or the passion to push through traditional boundaries and create innovative curriculums like Dr. Nerem. And most of us won't go back to school in our nineties like Nola Ochs. But we don't need to collect a Nobel Prize, publish a paper, start a program, or get a degree to develop our interests (see the box on page 81 for ideas). Learning and purpose find us far outside the classroom in our everyday lives. And the more we understand the deep connection between our purpose, learning, and health, the more we may optimistically grasp the pathways of education for all of us.

EXPAND YOUR TOOL KIT

Learning Your Purpose

No matter your age, your continual development as a human being matters to your health. Plus, the world needs your talents. What activities might help you to grow your interests and develop your creative voice? What have you always wanted to do but never made time for? Here are a few ideas to get you thinking about what captivates to you.

> Take a class or develop a skill such as photography, writing, cooking, dance, singing, piano, or hula. Read a book (nicely done!) or listen to how-to podcasts and put them into action. Notice when something captures your imagination. Keep a list. If a friend is also interested, invite her along.

> Visit your local library. It's incredible how a public library welcomes everyone and offers free classes and services. It's a great place to get away and gain a new perspective without ever leaving town. Plus, it can help you feel more connected to your community.[33]

> Many local universities allow older adults to audit classes. The Osher Lifelong Learning Institutes (based at Northwestern) partners with over 120 universities across the country, such as Duke, Northwestern, and UC Berkeley, to provide learning opportunities for people who are "50 or better."[34] (By the way, guess who their 2018 Keynote Conference Speaker was? Dr. Elizabeth Blackburn, of course.) Your local community center, library, and YMCA probably offer classes too.

> Check out online learning sites (Khan Academy, Udemy, Coursera, Open Culture, YouTube, etc.) that offer free or lower-

cost classes. An example is Yale University's most popular class ever, "The Science of Well-Being," by Professor Laurie Santos.

▸ Develop your own sense of purpose either through reflection, journaling, or volunteering for a cause that compels you. Action often fuels inspiration, rather than the other way around.

▸ If you are starting out in your career, please don't do things for the prestige alone or because someone else thinks it's a good idea for you. (I learned this the hard way.) Make sure you find genuine enthusiasm and meaning in the activities you say yes to. Say no to everything else. This will allow you time for the things that capture your imagination when they do arrive.

▸ Volunteer to help others unleash their potential too. This can range from offering to talk at a local elementary school about your work or tutoring kids after school at a local Boys & Girls Club. Whatever skills you have (and you have many; think broadly), consider sharing them with others. For instance, Airbnb has an Experiences program, where you can teach (or take) semiprivate lessons that range from surfing to milking a cow or attending concerts or events for social impact causes.[35] Have fun discovering niches you didn't even know you had!

Chapter Six

Neighborhood: Live and Play

Start where you are. Use what you have. Do what you can.
—ARTHUR ASHE

For my sixth birthday party, my parents hired a magician. In our cramped basement, Mr. Magnificent wowed the crowd with colorful handkerchief tricks and by pulling a white rabbit from a hat. For his final act, he called me to the front of the room. With the tap of a wand and a flash of his cape, he revealed a small round glass bowl with a beveled edge. It contained a present for me: one single goldfish.

Delighted by the big-eyed creature, I named him Snoopy. The next morning, I excitedly ran to the living room to see my new pet. I found Snoopy floating on his side, cause of death unknown. Like many party-favor goldfish, the festivities ended abruptly. To soothe my tears, my mom hugged me and said, "Honey, goldfish just don't live long. It was his time."

A couple of summers after Snoopy's untimely demise, my parents rented a Tudor-style vacation house in San Diego. The magical house came with indoor swings, an old tabby cat named Felicia, and an oversized concrete fishpond in the backyard. Felicia and I spent afternoons watching the large bright orange fish swirling the water in perpetual motion. Felicia, not a water lover by nature, couldn't resist dipping her paw in to bat at the lively creatures. The poker-faced fish moved out of the way, unfazed. Sitting beside the pond in California, I couldn't believe the magnificent, hardy animals living in the backyard were sickly Snoopy's cousins. Goldfish *could* thrive.

As it turns out, the widely shared assumption that all goldfish die young is an illusion. Goldfish can live twenty to thirty years. They can outlive most dogs and cats. According to the *Guinness Book of World Records*, the oldest recorded domestic goldfish, named Tish, died at forty-three years old in 1999. On that fateful day, he was set to rest in his owner's flower garden in a yogurt container. Tish and another fish called Tosh were a carnival prize awarded to a young British boy named Peter in 1956. Tosh died in 1976 at the age of twenty-two. Tish lived to see Peter move out of the house, get married, and have a mortgage. Peter's mom continued to care for Tish and chatted to him daily as a member of the family.[1]

In retrospect, Snoopy's untimely death after only one day had nothing to do with the average goldfish life span. Instead, the culprit seems something much more fundamental. Something important that Tish and Tosh had in common with the robust goldfish I met in California, and something Snoopy lacked. The fish that thrived had a rich environment. They weren't toted around in little plastic baggies only to end up trapped in a small party fishbowl. The Californian fish had an entire pond to play in, and Tish lived with caretakers who ensured his environment helped him thrive too. All living things must successfully navigate their environment to live. For a human being, that's our neighborhood.

Ben was a retired elementary school custodian in his late sixties with a kind smile, a soft voice, and snow-white hair. His wife, Sophie, had died of breast cancer four years before I saw him in our primary care residents' clinic. Ben and Sophie had been close companions, and Ben missed having Sophie to talk to over dinner and to accompany him on strolls in Central Park. In the years that Ben had lived alone in their apartment since Sophie's death, his metabolism had become out of whack. His blood glucose levels were out of control. He'd become extremely overweight and complained of bad knees. Ben lived in a second floor walk-up, and it took him fifteen minutes to get up and down the stairs. Now, without his wife at his side, it was difficult for him to get out and about. Ben's father was also severely overweight, and after going blind, he eventually died from complications relating to diabetes. Ben wondered if he'd inherited the family curse.

Ben patiently listened as I told him about the great opportunity to change his diet, eat more healthy green vegetables, and exercise more. At the time, it was my standard lifestyle lecture, passionately espousing the medical community's mantra of fewer calories and more exercise. It's the same tack that expensive public service campaigns take, aiming to teach people how to eat healthy. But at this point, don't we all know broccoli is better than a doughnut? When it comes to weight and health, there are hidden factors at play well beyond willpower alone.

When it comes to weight and health, there are hidden factors at play well beyond willpower alone.

If obesity is just about an individual's self-control or genetics, then it follows that expanded waistlines should be more or less evenly distributed. However, there's a curious gradient in towns across the country. For instance, in New York City, if you jump on the uptown C train at Spring Street in Soho, only about one in ten people in the neighborhood are obese. If you ride the train north in Manhattan about twenty minutes (6.7 miles) to West 125th Street in Harlem, the prevalence of obesity becomes one in four. Similarly, if you hop on the uptown 6 train on the Upper East Side at Ninety-Sixth Street, fewer than one in ten people are obese, but get off five miles north in the Bronx, where Ben lived, and the obesity rate jumps to one out of every three people. Even slight differences in location, like crossing Fourteenth Street, make a difference in weight.[2] Similar studies done in cities such as Boston and Chicago find similar dramatic differences within a tiny geographic radius.[3] It seems exposure to certain neighborhoods predicts pants size. Medically, this makes no sense. But if we consider neighborhoods in terms of the built environment and how many supermarkets and healthy food choices are easily accessible, we start to see how where we live can affect our waistlines.[4]

After I completed my lifestyle lecture, Ben told me he completely understood what I was saying. Mission accomplished! He then continued to explain that he wished he could eat healthier. The problem was, the closest food options to his apartment were a fried chicken joint and a small corner store that sold mostly soda, packaged foods, and cigarettes. Ben lived in a section of the Bronx that is a "food desert," where healthy options are scarce. The nearest grocery store was not within walking distance, and like a lot of New York subway stops, the closest to Ben didn't have a functioning elevator. Plus, even if he did manage to get himself to the grocery store, with his bad knees, he couldn't carry his groceries home. He didn't have anyone like Sophie to help him. With Ben's modest monthly pension, a regular taxi or delivery service didn't fit into his budget.

Food deserts contribute to "food insecurity," or not consistently having enough nutritious food to eat. In America in 2018, one in ten people, many of them children, regularly went hungry.[5] Thinking about food insecurity and hunger may conjure up a black-and-white Great Depression image of a gaunt individual in baggy clothes waiting in a food line. But the face of malnutrition in America today is Ben: a person with obesity standing in a fast-food line.[6]

The face of malnutrition in America today is Ben: a person with obesity standing in a fast-food line.

It may seem strange to equate the health of an obese person in America with a starving child abroad, but empty calories, just like insufficient caloric intake, create dietary deficiencies that hijack health. Studies of obese individuals reveal low micronutrients such as chromium, biotin, and thiamine. Micronutrients found in plant-based foods are essential to metabolic and immune functioning to ward off disease.[7]

Eating processed or fast food affects our health in other ways, too, ways that are just beginning to be understood through new, emerging research. A growing body of literature shows that eating whole plant-based foods, which our ancestors ate, is necessary for a healthy microbiome. This "neighborhood within" consists of trillions of symbiotic cells living mostly in our gut.[8] Whether you pick a salad or fries for lunch, you alter the composition of your gut microbes. And because different microbes process food differently, the composition affects your overall health and body in general.

Healthy versus unhealthy microbiomes also explain that frustration you might feel about a friend who eats chocolate with every meal and doesn't gain an ounce, while you seem to put on pounds with every lick of fat-free frozen yogurt. A study published in *Science* in 2013 blew my mind because it ran so counter to both common wisdom and what I'd learned in medical school. It showed that over time, genetically identical mice fed the exact same diet with the exact same number of calories became either lean or obese based on differences in gut flora alone.[9]

As a daughter, I recall my mom's constant struggles with her weight, even when counting calories, and the impact this had on her self-esteem. Over the years, I saw some of her well-meaning doctors make her feel worse. While shame and guilt around extra pounds are common, emerging science supports the idea that it's not just how many calories you eat, but where those calories come from that matters. Five hundred calories from a vegetable rice bowl aren't the same as five hundred calories from a greasy cheeseburger precisely because each feeds a different set of microbes in your gut. And the kicker is that a gut with healthy bacteria planted by healthy foods will handle the occasional cheeseburger—or doughnut—very differently than one fed a continuous diet of unhealthy fats and simple carbs. You and your friend really are processing that chocolate differently.

Even worse for our health and for those of us stuck with the limited selections of a corner store, the processed foods America depends on don't just make it hard to keep the weight off, they cause shifts in gut flora that weaken the microbiome and lead to a whole host of health problems. A sluggish microbiome can make us more prone to obesity, infections, inflammation, and neurocognitive disorders such as Alzheimer's and depression.[10] For now, there is no routine cheek swab or easy way to assess the composition of your microbiome, so all we can do is try to eat a diverse range of whole foods and vegetables. However, if you're intrigued, there are impressive crowdsourcing citizen-scientist collaborations, such as the large-scale American Gut Project (humanfoodproject.com/americangut/)

that will provide you with a personalized microbiome report in exchange for contributing deidentified data to science.[11]

So what can be done if we live in a food desert?

When it comes to diet, there are ways to bolster healthier food options.

One thing that could make a big difference is a weekly farmers' market. The brightly colored seasonal vegetables found at farmers' market stalls are often tastier, more nutritious, and cheaper than those sitting on a store shelf. There is a push nationally to ensure that people can use their food stamps at often less expensive farmers' markets.[12] Since the lack of competition in food deserts drives up store prices, introducing farmers' markets in food deserts can over time reduce local grocery store prices, which in one study decreased grocery bills about 12 percent in three years.[13] People also save money on travel when the market comes to them, which would have made a big difference for Ben, who couldn't travel easily. Plus, they are a great way to bring out the community, meet some neighbors, and support local businesses.

Community gardens can also help reduce food insecurity and provide an oasis in food deserts for at-risk schools and neighborhoods.[14] Studies show that if a child grows a vegetable, he or she is more likely to eat it.[15] A program in urban gardening in Colorado reports that three out of four students who participate in the school garden increase their produce consumption.[16] Also, community gardens provide physical activity for participants, beautify vacant lots or rooftops, and bring people together. School community gardens become outdoor classrooms and laboratories. Some schools even report that their community gardens boosted standardized test scores and reduced teacher turnover. Plus, the gardens provide summer jobs for high school students or others with barriers to employment, and business experience selling produce at local farmers' markets.[17] There's also evidence that community gardens and landscaping vacant lots significantly reduces gun violence in low-income neighborhoods.[18] It turns out a tomato is a powerful weapon.

Here's some more food for thought to boost access to healthy meals. The suggestions range from individual options to more ambitious partnerships. For instance, there are monthly delivery subscription services that specialize in local fruits and vegetables that are in season and thus a bit cheaper. You could talk to your corner store to see if stocking more fresh vegetables and fruits might be an option, and ask neighbors to chime in too. If you volunteer at a food pantry, see if there is a way to stock more than cans and include fresh fruit and vegetable donations. Consider forming a food co-op or partnering with a grocery store incubator program, such as in Detroit, Michigan. This model helps engage local citizens to address neighborhood food inequality. It boosts not only access to healthy meals but also local entrepreneurship.[19]

Our neighborhoods don't just determine what kinds of foods are easily available to us, they also influence how much exercise we get. My in-laws live in rural Ireland, and when I first visited, I imagined pleasant jaunts through the lush countryside, with perhaps a bleating sheep in tow. In reality, a walk there involves running from cars zipping along the narrow one-lane roads boxed in by stone walls. Without footpaths or sidewalks, it's unwalkable. For the modern worker seated at a computer for eight-plus hours a day, years on end, it's not easy to squeeze in the recommended daily fifteen thousand steps. It's even harder when you live in areas of urban sprawl or a sea of cul-de-sacs where shops are far from homes and driving is the norm and necessary. Walking's benefits are impressive: reducing the risk of headaches, cancer, depression, heart disease, arthritis, and osteoporosis. Meanwhile, sprawl is associated with a significant increase in chronic medical problems, such as high blood pressure and heart disease; it is the equivalent of aging the population by four years.[20]

Issues of inactivity are amplified when your street doesn't have connectivity through sidewalks. Studies from around the world show that the design of our neighborhoods substantially alters our physical activity.[21] The ability to get around a neighborhood easily on foot is known as "walkability." It's a hallmark of a healthy community. There are places to go and ways to easily get there by walking, which is particularly helpful for older people with mobility issues like Ben. Key features include aspects of the built environment like maintained even sidewalks, lights, traffic flow, shoulders, and crosswalks. You can find a restroom or take a break and rest when needed. Accessible public transportation is critical to connect walking areas as well. The benefits of walkability include support of local businesses, real estate property values, less noise pollution, and better air quality.

Activist Jane Jacobs, whose efforts prevented a freeway from cutting through Greenwich Village in Lower Manhattan, pointed out in her 1961 book *The Death and Life of Great American Cities* that there's a rhythm to city streets, which she called an "intricate ballet in which the individual dancers and ensembles all have distinctive parts which miraculously reinforce each other and compose an orderly whole." Sitting on a park bench in Washington Square in New York on a sunny weekday morning, it's a great joy to watch people crisscross the park to their destinations. Like the pleasant din in a busy café, the cacophony creates a whole. The daily dance may look random, but it's not. As behavioral economists and Starbucks know, people travel in predictable patterns. A city designed for walkability keeps the ballet in mind and amplifies rather than disrupts it.

More walkability and less traffic is better for health as well. We know this in part because of four days in December 1952, when a cold snap in London, England, suddenly caused fumes from burning coal to form a thick black smog that reeked like rotten eggs. In the days that followed, deaths spiked. In total, an estimated 12,000 people died and 150,000 more became ill.[22] The Great Smog of London established the clear association between increased fine particulate pollution levels in the air, such as from car exhaust and burning coal, and rates of cancers, heart disease, cognitive impairment, and death.[23] Health problems, including the risk of dementia, develop at levels far below the current guidelines for national air quality.[24] It seems women, children, and older adults are particularly at risk from neighborhood environmental pollutants.[25]

For instance, researchers using the large-scale Nurses' Health Study found a woman's risk of sudden cardiac death, which is unfortunately often the first symptom of heart disease for the victim, directly increased by proximity of her home to a major thoroughfare. I live by one, so this gave me pause. Those who lived closest (about 0.03 miles) to a major roadway had a 38 percent higher hazard of sudden cardiac death than those who lived even slightly farther away (about 0.3 miles) away. The association was linear, meaning that each tiny increment closer to a roadway increased the hazard. The study suggested that living in a home near a major roadway is potentially a greater risk to health than the known lifestyle risks of smoking, diet, or obesity.[26] Part of this may have to do with the noise, since noise pollution, from honks to sirens to garbage trucks at 4:00 a.m., is associated with impaired sleep, increased stress, worse mood, and health problems such as hypertension and heart disease.[27] (As I type this, I hear a jackhammer in the distance.)

Cities may be noisy and traffic-ridden, but they are often walkable and provide access to green spaces, which is critical. Wherever we live, taking time out in nature can provide a welcome respite. Plus, it's great for our health.

One early spring afternoon in 2015 I stood in the crisp air at a playground in Jackie Robinson Park in Harlem. Sunlight streamed through the tree branches, touching the chipped green paint of a swing set. Bird chirps broke up the city soundtrack, a mixture of chatter, sirens, and construction clanking. On assignment for an Urban Space and Health course at Columbia University, I visited the park in the previously disinvested district numerous times to understand how New Yorkers interacted with green space. I got to know the park in a way I hadn't done with other parts of the city. I observed the space and talked to the people using it: older women sitting on benches, teens playing basketball, and dog owners walking the perimeter. In the open air, I stayed open to possibilities.

My son Ryan, then five years old, often explored with me. After school, the A train took us 145 blocks north to Dunkin' Donuts. We'd sit in the window seat together, gobbling down pink frosted doughnuts with multicolored sprinkles before hitting the park. Walking to the park, we'd see men sitting and laughing together on stoops, pass the stores still with the bulletproof glass, and notice tourists holding guidebooks and talking in different languages at a recently opened coffee shop. One afternoon on the playground, Ryan made a friend. I watched the kids, one with white skin, one with brown, playing happily together below the new green buds on the trees. Two boys from different backgrounds and different parts of town delighted in the shared joy of the swings.

Green spaces connect us both physically and emotionally. Playgrounds, parks, and recreation centers provide a huge return both financially and on collective wellness. A prescription for a park may be in all our futures. Living in an urban area with more green space appears to improve overall well-being and reduce stress and headaches.[28] The longer participants stay and the more active they are, the greater the effect of the green space on well-being.[29] Do you live near a park? Shorter walking distances to green space from one's home correlate with improved mental health scores, even for people with diagnosed major depression.[30]

In addition, a study done in London showed that people living on streets with more trees had significantly lower rates of antidepressant prescriptions, even when controlling for income.[31] A large study of over ten thousand people in the UK over eighteen years found that the mental health boost from being near a park was equivalent to being married. In addition, greenery boosted neighborhood well-being even when there was poverty or high crime in the area.[32]

Spending time enjoying nature reduces cortisol levels, lowers blood pressure, and boosts immune function. Studies done in Japan measured salivary cortisol, heart rate, and blood pressure, and found that after walking in and observing a forest for about twenty minutes, participants had greater parasympathetic activity and lower sympathetic activity (in other words, they were less stressed). Other studies have collected blood and urine samples from men and women after they'd spent several days in nature, a practice known as *shinrin-yoku* or "forest bathing."[33] Compared to baseline levels from their day-to-day urban lives, the results showed that exposure to nature increased white blood cells known as "natural killer cells," which help fight off tumor growth and infection. The improved functioning extended for the month after the nature experience.[34]

Interestingly, you may not need a forest nearby to get a health boost from nature. A couple of trees may do. Researchers looked at about a decade of hospital data for the recovery wing of a surgical ward and found that patients whose hospital rooms looked out onto a patch of trees recovered a day sooner than those who looked out on a brick wall. They also needed less pain medicine and less encouragement from hospital staff.[35] Plants in the home helped reduce stress levels too.[36]

Just as a fish might be unaware of the water he lives in, we may be so immersed in our daily lives that we are unaware of environmental factors impacting our health. These are the "risk of risks." In other words, they are the underlying conditions that facilitate the advancement of diseases. And your neighborhood safety and sense of community is a big hidden factor.

Why is it so easy to miss the neighborhood connection to our health?

Partly because the connection between environmental factors and our health often shows up as vague physical symptoms. Take Daisy, our patient who appeared medically fine but felt too unwell to travel to see her favorite cousin, Viola. At Daisy's medical appointment, there was no clear trouble on a cellular, tissue, organ, or nervous system level. However, examining Daisy's life, she had much stress and heartache. And her neighborhood played a big role in these. In Brownsville, Brooklyn, where Daisy lived and where she grew up, she felt unsafe walking around at night on the dimly lit sidewalks with broken streetlights. Over time the area, once a cultural center of social activism, had become better known for street-corner drug dealing and homicides.[37] At night Daisy often heard gunshots in the distance. Once when she called the police to report a possible break-in at the building next door, they never came.

Over the years, Daisy knew many kids who died young from violence. She just never imagined one of them would be her teenage son. When Bryan, her only child, was alive, she worked hard to keep him focused on his schoolwork. But several years before I met her, Bryan was shot and killed during a robbery at the corner store where he'd stopped to buy a soda on his way home from band practice. Her community became a daily reminder of her grief and the loss of her child, who had meant everything to her.

In America, there is a reason that some neighborhoods—often just a subway or bus ride apart—are food deserts, less walkable, less safe, and more stressful. In 1933 Congress passed the Home Owners' Loan Act as part of the New Deal following the Great Depression. This act established the Home Owners' Loan Corporation, or HOLC (pronounced "Holk"), which created the opportunity for millions of Americans to avoid losing their homes by refinancing their mortgages with forgiving long-term loan packages.[38] At the time, banks foreclosed on more than one thousand homes a day nationally. At face value, the program sounds fantastic: more stability for more families. However, as is often the case, the devil's in the details.

To decide where to invest, HOLC, between 1935 and 1940, developed a simple classification system. Across nearly 250 American cities, the agency created maps with neighborhood ratings from A to D. The A neighborhoods, outlined on city maps in green, were considered desirable and a good investment. People in the A neighborhoods could get low-cost affordable loans to live the American Dream. Meanwhile, people asking for loans in the "hazardous" D neighborhoods, outlined on city maps in red, were ineligible. Their dreams deferred. No loan meant no opportunity for a family in a "redlined" neighborhood to leapfrog into a life of stable housing. It meant more stress and more price gouging by opportunistic landlords. It meant no playgrounds and parks for children. Documents available at the National Archives in Washington, DC, and an interactive online map created by historians depict the explicit criteria used by HOLC to determine the D rating: it plainly states, "Infiltration of: Negroes."[39]

The discriminatory practice of redlining based explicitly on race became the US Federal Housing Administration and real estate industry standard for decades following the New Deal. This formalized segregation was instituted across the country in every metropolitan area. Homeownership builds wealth and community, and redlining sparked a cycle of poverty that still impacts health decades later. For instance, the playground Ryan and I visited in Harlem was in a historically redlined district. Daisy's neighborhood, Brownsville, was once a redlined section of Brooklyn, which prevented people from getting legitimate loans for decades.[40] Years of underinvestment made these once vibrant neighborhoods unnecessarily unsafe and stressful to live in.

Daisy's neighborhood is far from the only section of a city or town in America where health outcomes vary by subway stop. For instance, in Chicago, at the Armitage stop in Lincoln Park, the infant mortality rate is 2.4 babies per 1,000 live births. If you get off at Garfield on the green line, less than ten miles away, the infant mortality rate is 19.3 babies per 1,000 live births, a rate worse than those in Ecuador, Iran, and Syria.[41]

Eight times the infant mortality in less than ten miles? This can't be explained by access to hospitals; world-class hospitals exist in all the cities that demonstrate this "subway effect." In addition, research suggests that medical care accounts for only 10 to 15 percent of preventable early deaths.[42] Instead, we have to look at our neighborhoods.

In America, a person's zip code is a stronger predictor of health than his genetic code. Although the distances between zip codes may be tiny, vast differences exist over a range of different health indicators: diabetes complications, strokes, deaths from heart disease, deaths from breast cancers, and premature babies.[43] For example, in 2016, the average life expectancy for a person in Washington, DC, was six years shorter than for a person living in bordering Montgomery County, Maryland (seventy-eight years versus eighty-four years).[44] The gap is amplified when taking skin color into account: the life expectancy of a black man in Washington, DC, is about twelve years less than that of a white man in Montgomery County (68.8 years versus 81.4 years).[45] That's the difference between two men dropping their granddaughters off to first grade on the same day and only one living to see her graduate from high school.

Living in a neighborhood where personal safety or the safety of loved ones is a constant concern also appears to accelerate telomere shortening. Dr. Katherine Theall and her colleagues measured the telomeres of ninety-nine children ages four to fourteen from a variety of neighborhoods around New Orleans, Louisiana. They found that kids from neighborhoods with high rates of unemployment, poverty, and "disorder," such as litter, broken glass, and boarded-up buildings, had three times the odds of having shorter telomeres than those living in more orderly and less stressful neighborhoods.[46]

The availability of nutritious food and walkability account for some of the difference. But that's not the complete story. Food inequality shows there are four times more supermarkets located in primarily white neighborhoods compared to neighborhoods of color.[47] And that Garfield subway stop in Chicago with the infant mortality rate eight times higher than the Armitage stop less than ten miles away? A 1939 HOLC map shows the area near Garfield clearly outlined in red. Where Ben lived in the Bronx, there was a similar story of structural disinvestment aggravated by the city's financial woes in the 1970s, with health effects of the stressful streets lasting decades later. And that structural disinvestment was driven by racism, a hidden factor we'll discuss further in chapter 7.

America is not alone in its social gradient of health. British epidemiologist Sir Michael Marmot and the World Health Organization have found unnecessary inequities in health around the world. The gradient is both between countries and within them. It exists between cities and within them. Neighborhoods only miles apart end up with health outcomes years apart.[48]

Much like the goldfish bowl, our neighborhoods are where we grow, live, age, play, and heal. For most of us, moving neighborhoods is impractical. We try to live in the nicest place we can afford that reflects what is important to us, urban or rural, bustling or laid-back. We must make do where we are. And there are plenty of things we can do to improve where we live even if we can't or have no desire to change locations.

While social, cultural, economic, and political choices shape our environment, we shape them too. At first glance, it may sound a bit intimidating to raise the larger structural changes our neighborhoods require to make them healthier places to live. But positive change is a part of neighborhoods too. And ideas are already flowing on what could be done.

The challenge is how to revitalize a neighborhood so people can take down the bulletproof glass and open cafés and stores without displacing the neighborhood's existing inhabitants. When gentrification replaces lower-income residents with higher-income inhabitants, there is risk of serial displacement, making the poor poorer.[49] In some cities, such as in Southwest Washington, DC, "zero displacement" campaigns have emerged to offset this.[50] City planners, urged by citizen's groups, are required to minimize the movement of existing residents in specific areas by creating a mix of market-rate and affordable housing. The goal is to help retain what makes a neighborhood unique while making it a safer, less stressful, and healthier place to live.

Neighborhoods are not fixed. And they don't exist in isolation. As Dr. Mindy Fullilove, a public psychiatrist who has done inspiring work on cities as a source of health and disease, says, "Geography is dynamic."

A city is like a living organism, and places change based on the choices people make. A single person has more power than she may realize. Dr. Fullilove continues, "A single individual can call a meeting."[51] Or plant some flowers. Or throw a party. Here is an opportunity each of us has to take action and improve health for everyone—and have something to look forward to in the process.

To make our neighborhoods feel less stressful and more like communities, we need to invest in each other. It's like the difference between a house and a home. Here is where ordinary citizen's groups play a powerful role in building connections and helping to reduce violence. New York University sociologist Patrick Sharkey found that residents and organizations within communities were a major reason for the massive twenty-five-year decline in crime in the US between 1990 and 2015. His research shows that neighborhoods with active community groups helped halve the homicide rate nationally. In cities with more than one hundred thousand people, every ten additional nonprofits led to a 9 percent reduction in the murder rate and a 6 percent drop in the violent crime rate.[52] This echoes other work such as in Philadelphia, where programs to fix up the exterior of abandoned buildings by removing trash, painting the facades, and securing the entrances lowered neighborhood gun violence by nearly 40 percent.[53] In addition, homes near "clean and greened" areas see a near 20 percent increase in property value.[54] Block associations, basketball programs, senior dance groups, community cleanups, after-school tutoring, music festivals: all of these play a role in improving neighborhood ties and neighborhood life. They make neighborhoods feel safer and more fun.

Dr. Fullilove and a team of volunteers in 2004 helped create Project CLIMB (City Life Is Moving Bodies) and the Giraffe Path in Upper Manhattan, an urban hike that unites seven parks spanning about six miles vaguely in the shape of a giraffe. The Giraffe Path cuts through previously redlined and disinvested communities in Harlem and Washington Heights where the crack epidemic in the 1980s escalated crime and decreased personal safety. Part of the idea for the hike came from seeing the dilapidated conditions in some of the neighborhood parks, such as broken stairways, uncleared paths, closed walking bridges, and rusty playground equipment. The idea was to bring attention to the parks and help connect physically close but historically isolated communities with an annual "Hike the Heights" ("Caminando los Altos") celebration.

On an unseasonably warm first Saturday in June, Ryan and I joined a diverse group of fellow hikers from all over New York City to wind along the Giraffe Path to a community potluck at the end. We walked a big section of the path with Maria, a woman in her seventies who had raised her children in Washington Heights and now participated in Hike the Heights every year with her kids and grandkids. As we entered the party in a sunken playground, fellow hikers greeted us with cheers, music, dancing, food, face painting, and papier-mâché giraffes made by local artists and children. The magic of the moment showed us that a neighborhood at its best isn't just a physical place, but a sense of community and connection.

> A neighborhood at its best isn't just a physical place, but a sense of community and connection.

Project CLIMB, along with the city parks department and the New York Restoration Project, literally is helping bridge neighborhoods with the 2015 reopening of the historic pedestrian High Bridge between Manhattan and the Bronx. In Brownsville, where Daisy lives, there is a homegrown effort to celebrate and improve the neighborhood, one creative idea at a time: from colorful murals to kale growing in urban gardens to the glimmer of community pride in the eyes of a child.[55]

And if you are new somewhere, you can create community too.

After a move from Boston to New York City, author Priya Parker and her husband, Anand Giridharadas, decided to start something called "I Am Here" days to get to know their new town.[56] The idea started with the two of them exploring the five boroughs for twelve hours at a time. Soon friends joined along. The ground rules include *unplug* (put aside technology and to-do lists), *commit* (stay for the whole adventure), *be present* (talk to the people you are with), and *be game* (come with a spirit of adventure and expect surprises). And, of course, have respect for the neighborhood being visited.

On their travels, they've wandered into shops, cafés, synagogues, daytime dance parties, and conversations. They've admired graffiti, art museums, and nude sculptures. They've eaten new foods, tried new beers, and seen New York with fresh eyes. If you're inspired to try something similar in your city, check out their #IamHere Days blog for inspiration and logistics.[57]

Recognizing your entire city is all part of the same community and fostering connections is the foundation of hidden health. Plus, it's fun.

Just like my ill-fated goldfish, Snoopy, as humans, we are often put into environments that we have little control over, at least initially. Yet where one lives affects health profoundly. Our neighborhoods are one of the most important yet well-hidden factors in our health. They influence our waistlines, expectations, opportunities, security, mental health, and life span. Western medicine remains focused on the hope that biomedical advances will cure diseases such as cancer, heart disease, and hypertension. Meanwhile, mountains of public health data suggest we can align our daily choices and environments to contribute to the main predictors of health, starting with focusing on our neighborhoods.[58] As Dr. Fullilove says, "Take one step, and the rest will follow."

As we'll see next, it's not just where we live and play that makes a healthy community, it's also how we treat each other.

Live and Play

Take a moment to think about where you live and your neighbors. What makes it feel like a community? How might you develop more of a sense of ownership and connection to where you live?

> Look around your neighborhood and imagine how to beautify it. Care for it like it is a living thing. Pick up three pieces of trash a day, plant flowers, paint over graffiti, organize the painting of a mural, or post a sign that offers a positive message to passersby.

> Seek out farmers' markets and support community gardens. If you have time or a green thumb, volunteer. If you want to organize one for your neighborhood, think about what existing community groups and businesses you might partner with. Check out the University of Florida's step-by-step guide to starting a farmers' market to get ideas.[59]

> Spend time in nature. It's good for both physical and mental health. If you can't go out, bring nature to you. Buy a plant or give one. (Ultimate bonus points if you grew it yourself or built the pot in a pottery class!) Take joy in caring for it. If you have kids or grandkids, involve them.

> Cultivate your local communal green spaces, such as parks, walkways, bike lanes, or patios. If greenery is lacking, consider how it might be added. If there is a vacant or trash-filled lot, get some neighbors or local businesses together to help clean and landscape it. Involve neighborhood kids. Teach others how trees and grass boost neighborhood safety.

> In the "killing two birds with one stone" category, start a parent/child community service group with other local parents. As one mom who did this noted, "Community and community service all in one fell swoop."

> Celebrate the positive things in your community (like that newly landscaped lot or a special bit of history) that uplifts people. Throw a party or parade. Introduce yourself to new neighbors. Enlist the knowledge of seniors in your neighborhood who have seen it transform over time.

> If you see a person on the street asking for money, offer her a snack or water. Ask her name. If you don't have anything, acknowledge her request and tell her you wish you could help. You may be the only kind person she encounters today. If a person looks unwell, ask if she is okay, or if she needs you to call for help. (ERs are required to see patients regardless of their ability to pay.) If it's a nonemergency, see if your city has a help line you can call to alert them to someone in need.

> Notice your travel patterns in your city, where you go and where you don't. Cross the street and branch out. Try out a new route to work or the store so you can see your neighborhood with fresh eyes. Consider visiting a new public library or playground or dog park or café to explore your hometown. Search out "the best" pizza slice or cup of coffee or pancakes and see where the search leads you. Bring along a friend or your child to make it an afternoon adventure. Make a point of talking to the people you meet along the way.

> If you have a pet fish, please get it an adequate-size bowl. And learn how to prep the water so it can thrive. RIP, Snoopy.

Chapter Seven

Fairness:
Living by the Golden Rule

Where, after all, do universal human rights begin? In small places, close to home—so close and so small that they cannot be seen on any maps of the world. Yet they are the world of the individual person; the neighborhood he lives in; the school or college he attends; the factory, farm, or office where he works. Such are the places where every man, woman, and child seeks equal justice, equal opportunity, equal dignity without discrimination. Unless these rights have meaning there, they have little meaning anywhere.

—ELEANOR ROOSEVELT

In my third year of medical school, senior surgeon Dr. Quintus Mack stood imposingly, with his perfectly combed hair and pressed white coat, at the front of the small group of students. Nimble in the Socratic method, he fired a series of questions at us about various procedures and medical conditions. In rapid succession, he called on my classmates. Every question Dr. Mack asked, I answered correctly in my head. I predicted the follow-up questions too. My excitement grew, like a contestant on a game show about to win the cruise to Jamaica. I felt unstoppable. My long hours of study were set to pay off.

Only I never got asked the questions.

The entire teaching session, Dr. Mack never made eye contact with me or acknowledged any of the several women in the group. I felt my face grow hot with disappointment and anger. The next meeting repeated the pattern. My frustration became intolerable. After all, Dr. Mack's feedback helped determine our grade, and our grades governed residency prospects. Friends who had finished the rotation said not to take the slight so personally. "Everyone knows he ignores the women. He's done it forever."

His treatment of the women students gnawed at me any time I thought about the clerkship. Many times, I imagined what I'd say if I saw him again. And then, years later, the opportunity presented itself when I bumped into him at a cocktail party. Instead, we chatted about his golden retriever, Molly. As we talked, I realized he wasn't a terrible person, or even blatantly sexist. He spoke proudly of his wife's new novel and the fact that his daughter had decided to major in engineering. I began to rationalize his behavior. Maybe it was a generational thing, and he didn't want to put the women on the spot? When I gathered my courage and brought up the clerkship, he seemed surprised and oblivious of his unequal treatment.

Being treated as invisible in our day-to-day lives isn't just annoying. It has significant implications for our careers—and our health. We know from research discussed in chapter 4 that there is a physical link between our status at work and our bodies. Which means a lot of us out there are at risk. For instance, the pervasive gender gap in the workplace starts early, especially in the sciences and academics.[1] It still makes my ears burn when I remember how a department chair at a major hospital told me he would hire more women for leadership roles if there were just "more qualified women out there." I wanted to shout, "But there are!" The problem is that it's easy to overlook qualified people when they don't fit the current mold.

Yale researcher Jo Handelsman published a clever experiment in 2012 to demonstrate this point. She gave 127 male and female professors across six universities two identical CVs and asked them to evaluate the "applicants" for a laboratory manager position. The only difference was that one applicant was named Jennifer and the other John. Professors of both genders equally rated Jennifer as less competent and offered her fewer job and mentoring opportunities. And to top it off, Jennifer was offered $3,730 less pay per year than John for the same position.[2] Even people in science who pride themselves on objectivity are at risk of bias.

Bias extends beyond gender differences, particularly with race and ethnicity. Studies have found that an African American man without a criminal record is less likely to get interviewed for a job than a white man with a criminal record.[3] Another study found whiter-sounding names like Emily or Greg increased the odds of being called back for an interview over names such as Lakisha or Jamal, even on identical résumés.[4] Other research from 2011 shows that when a typical white-sounding name or a typical Arab-sounding name was affixed to two similar résumés, the Arab male applicant needed to send out two résumés for every one résumé sent by a white male applicant for a callback.[5] Researchers found that having a white-sounding name was the equivalent of adding eight years of experience to a CV.[6] Unchecked individual bias collectively creates institutional discrimination.

> Unchecked individual bias collectively creates institutional discrimination.

And that institutional discrimination creates pay gaps. In 2016 the US Census Bureau found full-time, year-round jobs across numerous professions pay women about 80 cents for every dollar a man makes in the same position.[7] According to the Pew Research Center, over her career, a woman would need to work five to six years more to make the same amount as a man, still leaving her with less money in retirement.[8] The pay gap is far worse for women of color, with estimates showing that for every dollar a white male worker makes, a black woman earns from 47 to 69 cents.[9] In New York City, according to the comptroller's office, to attain the same earnings as her white male counterpart, she would need to work an additional thirty years.[10]

Some attribute the pay gap to career patterns, saying women are more likely to take time off or scale back with family. However, the gap is even higher for female professionals at the top of their fields, from corporate executives to academic department chairs to Oscar-nominated actresses.

In 2017 it came to light that for reshoots of the film *All the Money in the World*, the actress Michelle Williams was paid less than 1 percent of what her male costar Mark Wahlberg received for the same days of work. Wahlberg was paid $1.5 million, and Williams got about $1,000, which worked out to $80 a day.[11]

This discrepancy is not an isolated case. When studies control for education and experience across fields, the gender pay gap remains. In 2018, at the current rate of incremental change, the gender gap in the US will close in forty-three years, about the time my now ten-year-old son Max is starting to think about retirement. And some places lag further behind.[12] In Wyoming—where the state motto is "Equal Rights," since it was the first to give women the vote—it will take an estimated 136 years for the gender pay gap to close.[13] By then, my great-great-granddaughter will be nearing retirement.

Something I did not initially understand is that a "pay gap" is a "health gap" in disguise. Advocating for fairness in pay is advocating for better health. For decades, doctors have noticed that women are far more prone to depression and anxiety than men. Studies show the prevalence of depression and anxiety in women is about twice the prevalence of those same mood disorders in men, starting in adolescence and persisting across the life span.[14]

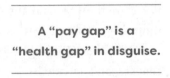

A "pay gap" is a "health gap" in disguise.

Yet, suspiciously, the search for hormonal or biological markers that predispose women to depression hasn't yet yielded a clear culprit. Some of the difference may be due to the underdiagnosis of depression in men. But emerging evidence suggests the main reason for the discrepancy may rest more in our wallets than our brains.

A study done at Columbia University looked at the relationship between mood disorders and the gender pay gap. The researchers used data from a survey of 22,581 working adults to find the effects of gender discrimination, as reflected through income differences, on mood disorders. They found that women who were paid less than equally qualified men had about two and a half times the risk of depression and four times the risk of anxiety. Even after controlling for differences in age, occupation, education, and family structure, the findings remained. Meanwhile, among women who were paid equally to the men, there was no increased risk of depression or anxiety.[15] The wage gap study and others like it suggest that the greater numbers of women with mood disorders may reflect a social inequity, not an underlying biological cause. The findings are also consistent with data showing that societies with less economic inequality have better health outcomes.[16]

> Women who were paid less than equally qualified men had about two and a half times the risk of depression and four times the risk of anxiety.

Equal pay for equal work is a health issue, but when was the last time you saw a doctor for a salary checkup?

So to maximize women's health, what if men and women swapped places in the workplace? Not so fast. In an ironic twist, the economic system that seems to favor men in the short term may be responsible for those men's undoing in the long term. In developed nations, including the United States and the United Kingdom, men have higher rates of mortality across all ages, on average dying nearly seven years earlier than women. These findings include all causes of death from heart disease, cancers, and suicide.[17]

The current medical model implies health outcomes have different underlying genetics. Something about male bodies (testosterone levels are often deemed the culprit) predisposes men to live shorter lives. Yet population studies reveal the risk of premature death might be more about our culture than our biology. High levels of patriarchy, or gender inequality, in a society correlate with an increased all-cause mortality among men.[18] The more egalitarian the community, such as an Israeli kibbutz, the more males are likely to live as long as females.[19] Perhaps the "weathering" effect of a high daily allosteric load (stress),

> A more egalitarian culture is less stressful for everyone and promotes better health outcomes for women and men.

the net effect of the economic burdens that overwhelmingly fall to men, leads to premature aging and death.[20] Evidence suggests a more egalitarian culture is less stressful for everyone and promotes better health outcomes for women and men.[21] So how do we let our individual biases get in the way?

Bias is a preconceived opinion that influences thoughts, feelings, and behaviors. It takes different forms. The most obvious is *explicit bias*, which is a conscious attitude about a group of people. While sometimes it can seem artificially positive—like thinking women are more nurturing than men, or that Asian students are good at math—it's an overt stereotype. Explicit bias or prejudice can be in-your-face: a swastika on a children's playground, a noose in front of an African American history museum, or a "No Gays Allowed" sign in a hardware store window. Explicit bias is blatant discrimination or hate: sexism, racism, homophobia, transphobia, xenophobia, anti-Semitism, or Islamophobia. While individuals play a role, discriminatory Jim Crow laws, policies, and practices also fuel explicit bias.[22]

Implicit bias, otherwise known as *unconscious bias,* on the other hand, is a more intuitive automatic attitude or behavior.[23] The stigma seen with implicit bias can contradict a person's conscious spoken beliefs, which makes it tricky. It makes you wonder, *Did that just happen? Am I being overly sensitive?* Or, *Seriously???* It sneaks up as slights in everyday experiences: at work, in class, at an interview, at a bar with colleagues, while shopping, looking for a restroom, or even at the doctor's office. The thought that something isn't right gnaws at you. It's the subtle behaviors and social tics that hint at unconscious attitudes. *He's acting like I'm naive.* Or, *Is he making fun of me?* Or, *Is she scared of me?* The person with the implicit bias is often unaware of their actions, which may contradict explicit spoken beliefs.

Implicit bias creeps into hospitals too.

Professionalism is the cornerstone of medicine. It is an obligation of the calling to use knowledge and skills for the benefit and healing of all patients in need.[24] Being a doctor means striving to treat all patients with equity even in challenging situations. But just as health occurs in a context, so too does education. Medical students of all backgrounds may learn something unexpected from their training: how to treat patients differently. Research by Harvard psychiatrist Dr. Edward Hundert shows that much of what students learn in medical school is from the informal "hidden curriculum," unintended daily lessons that convey an unspoken culture.[25] In other words, an eye-roll can teach more than a PowerPoint presentation.

There is a vast amount of data about how physician bias affects doctor-patient interactions. Studies show that when a physician holds an implicit bias toward his patients, he may act more authoritarian, dominate the conversation more, engage a patient less in decisions about her medical care, or provide substandard care.[26] For example, a study in the *New England Journal of Medicine* found doctors manage chest pain differently based on race and sex, even though, medically speaking, there's no reason for it.[27] Notably, the odds of a physician referring a black woman for a cardiac treatment were 40 percent less than for a white man.

Bias can manifest as acts of omission as well. For instance, researchers found that a patient with a same-sex partner often isn't asked routine health screening questions.[28] Or a patient with high-functioning autism may not get listed as eligible for the organ transplant list, even though autism is not a criterion for exclusion.[29] A patient who speaks a language other than English may have her care delayed while English speakers who arrived later are seen first. Stigma about obesity in medical settings makes obese people less inclined to seek medical care.[30] Bias toward people with mental illness remains a major barrier to medical care as well.[31]

In addition, people of color are overdiagnosed with mental illness. African Americans are four times more likely than white patients to receive a diagnosis of schizophrenia.[32] And there is not a shred of decent evidence that this is due to underlying genetics. It probably has more to do with hidden factors in our society and that the criteria for disorders is applied unevenly across skin colors. So, for example, a clinician's unconscious bias may lead her to underdiagnose mood disorders such as bipolar disorder for an African American patient and overdiagnose a psychotic disorder such as schizophrenia. It seems a subtle sense of "other" tinkers with doctors' thinking. Some researchers speculate that unconscious bias plays a role in why a patient of color is more likely to die in the hospital after a traumatic injury.[33] His symptoms may not get the benefit of the doubt, and critical signs are often dismissed.

As a medical intern, I had a patient in his forties admitted with pancreatitis. Originally from Bangladesh, Omar worked as a cabdriver and sent money to his family back home. Every morning when my team arrived in Omar's room on our rounds, he'd writhe in pain and tell us he was dying. But the nursing staff reported that when we left and he thought no one was watching, he looked comfortable watching TV. Our impression was that he was overreacting and "med seeking." He perceived that we weren't willing to help him and became increasingly hostile in return. Because his behavior was so unpleasant, we avoided extra visits to his room. We'd run out of time for his afternoon check-in. Eventually, I became just as dismissive of his complaints as my colleagues. Several days into his stay, the nurse on the morning shift found him in his room, dead. There was no family we could reach to request an autopsy. Many years later, I still think about what we missed and all that went unsaid. How had bias played a role in his death?

Navigating daily bias at work or while driving a car or just trying to grab a snack at the mini-mart is stressful. In the 1970s Harvard psychiatrist Dr. Chester Pierce wanted to study the daily slights and nonverbal put-downs that people of color experience. To describe these subtle everyday instances of racism, he coined the term *microaggressions*. Unfortunately, Dr. Pierce knew discrimination well. As an undergraduate at Harvard University, he played tackle at the first integrated football game in 1947 at the University of Virginia. At that historic event, he had to sleep in a separate dorm from his white teammates.[34] Dr. Pierce hypothesized that daily slights, over time, added up to adverse health outcomes. A kind of death by a thousand cuts.

Columbia University professor and multicultural scholar Dr. Derald Wing Sue furthered Dr. Pierce's early work. As a child of parents who emigrated from China to Portland, Oregon, Dr. Sue was teased by other kids for his ethnicity while he was growing up in the 1950s. As a psychology student, he began to study how prejudice perpetuates.[35] His research uncovered an array of "brief and commonplace daily verbal, behavioral, or environmental indignities, whether intentional or unintentional."[36] These usually fall into the categories of microassaults, microinsults, and microinvalidations. Dr. Sue's work helped inspire a popular blog started by Columbia University students called MicroAggressions.com, which makes "visible the ways in which social difference is produced." The goal is to form "connections between our everyday interactions" with "larger systems."[37] In other words, we all play a role.

Here's a scenario. Ahmad is a young man routinely asked by people he introduces himself to, including teachers and professors, where he's from. When he says, "Here," they respond, "No, originally." A writer who is Asian American feels she's developed a "sidekick complex" after never seeing a movie or reading a book starring an Asian American superhero. In workplace diversity training, a man who identifies as gay shares with his group that the word *homosexual* is offensive to him. A straight participant disagrees.[38] While each incident by itself may seem relatively minor, when taken side by side, they show the bigger picture of prejudice. Like Magic Eye posters from the 1990s, after you stare at a random pattern for long enough, suddenly a 3-D shark pops out. Microaggressions, taken together over time, create macroaggressions.

Microaggressions, taken together over time, create macroaggressions.

Time would prove Drs. Pierce and Sue correct. The day-to-day hassles of living in a culture where you feel threatened, harassed, or disrespected take a toll on the body. Individuals who report experiencing discrimination have higher rates of disease. It leads to chronic activation of the hypothalamic-pituitary-adrenocortical (HPA) axis, cortisol levels, cytokines, glucose levels, and blood pressure reactivity with a cascade of health problems such as stroke, cancers, and heart disease.

The hidden health tax of discrimination can also significantly impact offspring. After the Twin Tower attacks on September 11, 2001, people in the US who were perceived as Arab Americans experienced increased harassment and violence as backlash. In a remarkable study, researchers interested in the effects of social discrimination on health looked at California birth certificates from the six months following 9/11 compared to the same six calendar months one year earlier. What they found was striking. Women with Arabic-sounding names were a third more likely to give birth to a low-birth-weight baby than they were the year prior. Low birth weight is associated with a host of health problems later in life.[39] The risk increased further if the child had a distinctive Arabic name, which suggested a stronger ethnic identification and potentially increased discrimination. No other group was affected.[40] Undoubtedly not all the women experienced harassment directly, but the cultural shift seems to have seeped into the womb. Whether because of religious, racial, economic, gender, sexual orientation, or immigration status, feeling unwelcome puts people at risk of poorer health.

I like to think I make up my own mind about people and situations. Popular opinion sways other people, but not me. Yet a growing body of evidence challenges this notion and suggests we all walk around with blind spots. Researchers Anthony Greenwald (University of Washington), Mahzarin Banaji (Harvard University), and Brian Nosek (University of Virginia) study social cognition, the thoughts and feelings outside of one's conscious awareness. Together, they figured out a way to test for hidden biases. The idea is that recognizing secret opinions lurking deep in the brain is the first step to keeping them in check.

The researchers developed a standardized quiz called the Implicit Association Test (IAT) that is available for free online. In fewer than ten minutes, you're shown a series of words or pictures and given seconds to sort them into simple categories as quickly as possible. It's not long enough to think—only to make a snap decision. The test is scored based on how long it takes you to associate positive and negative words with the subject, such as black and white faces.

The IAT can't predict an individual's behavior, but it's a good springboard for discussion. The test is simple, but challenges our presumptions about the kinds of people we are. Before taking the exam, there is an ominous hard-stop prompt. The user must click a button that accepts the following statement: "I am aware of the possibility of encountering interpretations of my IAT test performance with which I may not agree." We may believe we are unbiased, but our keystrokes show something different. It seems everyone has unconscious bias. Young or old, student or teacher, Democrat or Republican, research shows we all share implicit bias. No one is immune.

While bias is part of being human, it seems even artificial intelligence (AI) can act like Uncle Marty after a few margaritas. For example, software engineers working on automated language systems, such as Google Translate, must regularly intervene to reduce unintentional bias. Left to their own algorithms, AI systems are more likely to associate male pronouns with words such as leader, boss, director, doctor, programmer, and president and female pronouns with words like assistant, helper, employee, nurse, coworker, and teacher. Researchers have caught AIs pairing women with housework and making grossly stereotypical age and ethnic assumptions, such as associating the terms *Mexican* and *illegal*. The thing is, an automated machine isn't racist or a sexist pig. It's just synthesizing the vast subjective bias conveyed in hundreds of billions of words on the internet. It's learning from us.

In my public health training, I took a series of IATs with eye-opening results. For a blond-haired, blue-eyed woman who grew up partly in the racially divided American South, I was surprised to see that I did not show racial or ethnic bias on several tests. While that does not give me a free pass, it was reassuring.

Then, as the warning predicted, came the cognitive dissonance. It is still ringing in my ears. On the gender test, I showed not a slight bias, but a *moderate* bias linking female with family and male with career, which contradicts my firm, outspoken feminist beliefs. It also runs contrary to my history: my dad was my primary caretaker while my mom worked outside the home. Now I have a family and career of my own, and I love that my husband is an equal partner. So when I saw my findings, I was stunned. Undoubtedly it was an error. So I retook it—twice—and got similar results. A related test concluded something similar. How could such a discrepancy exist?

It's not necessarily comforting, but I'm not alone in my unconscious gender bias. Half of people who take the IAT moderately or strongly associate women with family and men with career. Conversely, 2 percent of respondents moderately or strongly associate the opposite: men with family and women with career. Even with a margin of error, this is statistically significant. Did I drink the cultural Kool-Aid and unknowingly internalize gender bias?

Odds are, that's exactly what happened. As Gloria Steinem said, "You could not subordinate half the human race unless some of that was internalized." It seems when society repeatedly sends a message that you're supposed to be a certain way, it's hard not to receive it deep down in your brain. It's like a subliminal fast-food ad in the middle of your favorite TV show. Or a neurologic patient with cortical blindness who catches a ball he can't see. We absorb the culture around us, sometimes unknowingly.

During a trial in 1952 that would eventually become the testimony for *Brown v. Board of Education*, Dr. Kenneth Clark, a well-respected New York psychologist, took the stand. The lawyers, whose team included future Supreme Court justice Thurgood Marshall, asked the mild-mannered scholar to explain to the court the "doll experiment." A lawyer for the defense recounted later that at first he thought the request was a joke. Dr. Clark explained that he had designed the study with his wife, Dr. Mamie Clark.[41]

To pause for a moment, it's hard to overstate how accomplished and groundbreaking the Clarks were. They were remarkable scholars and leaders. Among their many achievements, they were the first and second African Americans to earn doctorates in psychology at Columbia University, in 1940 and 1943, respectively. The Clarks were early proponents of emotional intelligence and "training for kindness without apology." In a 1984 television interview, long before AI, Dr. Kenneth Clark said, "one of the most dangerous things facing mankind today is a use and training of intelligence excluding moral sensitivity."[42] They paved the way for much of the research presented in this chapter.

In the doll experiment, boys and girls of color, ages six to nine, were shown two identical baby dolls. The only difference was that one had dark skin and one had light skin. A researcher asked the child a series of questions about how he or she felt about the dolls. When asked which doll looked "nice," child after child pointed at the white one. When asked which doll was "bad," they pointed at the black one. The final question the researchers asked the child was which doll looked "like you."

At the trial, Dr. Carter explained why he asked each child the questions in a particular order. "I wanted to get the child's free expression of his opinions and feelings before I had him identify with one of these two dolls." In films of the experiment, which researchers have replicated many times over, it is heartbreaking to watch any child identify a doll as the "bad one" and then, with the point of a finger and a glance, also acknowledge that doll looks like him. I lose my breath every time.

Dr. Clark noted that a "child accepts as early as six, seven or eight the negative stereotypes about his own group." He warned, "Human beings who are subjected to an obviously inferior status in the society in which they live, have been definitely harmed."[43] They adopt the message that their value is less. This is known as *internalized bias*. In a concrete example of this devaluation, in a 2011 blog post, *Freakonomics* author Stephen Dubner noted the results of his online search for a toy called "My First Dollhouse." If the house came with a "Caucasian family," it was $64. The price of the same house with an "African American family" was $38. While the reasons for the discrepancy are not clear, since they were different sellers, it is nevertheless disheartening.[44] After all, 2010 follow-up research to the Clarks' doll studies showed that children of all skin tones preferred playing with the white dolls.[45] Data from the IAT shows roughly 70 percent of people, including many people of color, have an unconscious preference for white over black skin.[46]

Internalized bias has real-world health consequences. For instance, research reveals that people with high internalized bias against their group show biologic changes, such as increased rates of glucose intolerance, obesity, and depression.[47] They are also more likely to drink alcohol excessively.[48] Also, a study of ninety-two African American men between the ages of thirty and fifty looked at the interaction between high internalized bias and real-world discrimination. People who were most often experiencing discrimination at work, in trying to find housing, and out in public, as well as having high internalized bias, had significantly shorter telomeres.[49] Biologically speaking, they were 1.4 to 2.8 years older than their actual age. Interestingly, those with high discrimination but low internalized bias—in other words, a more positive self-image—did not seem to have shorter telomeres.

Internalized bias can also impact the quality of health care a person receives. According to a Harvard study, doctors with a high level of unconscious bias against black people are less likely to treat black patients.[50] There is even ample evidence that doctors who are black can hold a negative bias toward black patients.

Feeling like you don't belong can influence behavior in insidious ways. In the early 1990s psychologist Dr. Claude Steele tried to figure out why black students at the University of Michigan underperformed and dropped out at higher rates than their white peers. Between high school grades and SAT scores, the students looked similar on paper. But in practice, Dr. Steele knew there was a 25 percent greater risk of a student of color dropping out of school. He suspected hidden cultural factors made the black students feel unwelcome and unconsciously hijacked their performance.

To foster a sense of community and acceptance, Dr. Steele and his colleagues designed a "living and learning" community for 250 racially diverse first-year students transitioning to college life. The program offered weekly academic support and "rap groups" to talk about the transition. At the end of the study, the black students in the program not only had better first-year grades than black students not in the program, but they also didn't underperform compared to white students. In other words, it seemed a sense of belonging in the groups caused the major outcome differences to evaporate. There were not innate differences between the black and white students, but environmental triggers with a measurable effect on behavior and performance.[51]

In an ingenious follow-up experiment, which has been replicated hundreds of times in different ways, Steele and his colleagues tested black and white students on the verbal section of the GRE. He told one group the test measured intelligence and the other group that it did not reflect intellectual ability. When the exam was labeled an "intelligence test," the black students performed worse than white students. When it was not, they did equally well.[52] He called this phenomenon *stereotype threat*, when a person unintentionally acts in the way others perceive him as a self-fulfilling prophecy. Not just race but also ethnicity, gender, sexual orientation, and social standing can trigger stereotype threat.[53]

For example, research shows a woman will underperform on a math test if something reminds her that she is female before the test. For women taking a calculus exam, just ticking a box with one's gender before the exam versus afterward led to a sizable drop in women's scores. Conversely, if told beforehand that women typically perform better on the exam, females' scores go up. A *stereotype boost*. The same applies to students of color. It seems all students, including white male students, perform worse if they believe they are somehow part of an inferior group before taking the exam, or better if they think they're part of a select group. A small reminder of a negative or positive stereotype before a task "primes" the brain for what follows.[54] One strategy that's inferred from this data: If you fear you face discrimination, before you go into a test or situation, remind yourself of being a part of a smaller group or a club (i.e., a math club, an honor society, etc.) that does well on this exam or in this situation. It doesn't hurt to try, and it may help.

Here's how the brain gets flummoxed with stereotype threat. Trying to interpret a negative stereotype uses mental energy. It's sort of like leaving a bunch of apps running in the background on your smartphone. The distraction hijacks working memory.[55] The extra effort to ignore or disprove a stereotype distracts from focusing 100 percent on the task at hand. Fatigue increases. Performance declines. It seems so unfair.

Similar to what Dr. Pierce, the Harvard University researcher who looked at everyday racism, hypothesized, conscious or unconscious awareness of one's group identity impacts biology in strange ways. For instance, studies show that when stereotype threat activates for African American males, such as when a test is labeled a test of intelligence, anxiety increases and blood pressure rises.[56] If prolonged, high blood pressure puts people at risk for cardiovascular disease. But someone who's black and living in America may negotiate stereotype threat in the form of microaggressions throughout the day.

The Study of Women's Health Across the Nation (SWAN) examined everyday discrimination such as feeling treated with less courtesy and less respect, and receiving poorer service. The study found that black women who reported high levels of daily discrimination had more serum markers of inflammation and higher rates of subclinical carotid artery disease.[57] This picture calls into question long-standing assumptions in the medical community that black patients are biologically more prone to hypertension.

So how do we explain this? Here is what we know. In the United States, a black infant has twice the mortality rate of a white baby. Records from 2015 show this gap has remained persistent over time.[58] The hidden factors of neighborhoods, education, and income play roles in this health disparity. However, there is more to the story: data shows the child of a middle-class, college-educated black woman is slightly more likely to die before her first birthday than the child of a white woman living in poverty with less than a college education.[59] And this mysterious health gap persists over time. After all, the life expectancy of a black child born in 2015 is 3.5 years shorter than that of a white child (see figure 3).

Some argue that the gap in health outcomes is due to some underlying genetic differences in race that account for differences in disease. But the more we learn about genetics, the more this argument doesn't hold up.

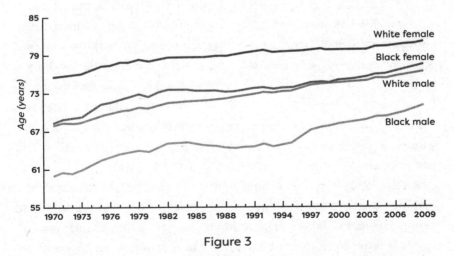

CDC LIFE EXPECTANCY GRAPH AT BIRTH, BY RACE AND SEX

Figure 3

Elizabeth Arias, "United States Life Tables, 2009" (2014), US Department of Health and Human Services, Centers for Disease Control and Prevention, National Center for Health Statistics (accessed December 18, 2018), https://www.cdc.gov/nchs/data/nvsr/nvsr62_07.pdf.

For example, health disparities evaporate if others classify a person of color as "white," even if that's not how the person of color self-identifies. In other words, a person who "passes as white" gains a significant health advantage. It seems the health disparity may reflect an internalization of cultural bias more than unique biology.

In an experiment done as part of the PBS series *RACE: The Power of an Illusion*, students in a DNA workshop predicted they'd have similar genetics to others in their group who had similar skin color. The results showed no significant genetic correlation based on skin color, as have many subsequent studies.[60] Humans, after all, are about 99.9 percent genetically similar.[61] Dr. Anita Foeman leads the DNA Discussion Project at West Chester University in Pennsylvania, where she asks students to draw out what they think their ancestry is; participants are often shocked by the mismatch in their personal identity and their actual genetic results.[62] Many people are now discovering this in their own homes after receiving unexpected ancestry results from commercially available DNA testing kits.

Medicine has historically mistaken social differences for underlying genetic differences. But aside from skin color, there are no consistent genetic markers that define race. In other words, black and white are meaningless under a microscope. Genotype, or what the genes contain, defies phenotype, or how a person looks. Two individuals with the same skin color may have less genetically in common than two people with different skin colors. Advances in genetics reinforce that "race" is a social construct rather than a biological one.

> **Medicine has historically mistaken social difference for underlying genetic differences.**

In the 1920s in the US several southern states declared that if a child had "one drop" of "black blood," he was black. If the same child moved from Virginia to Maryland, he suddenly became white. Similar confusing definitions have been used with people of Native American ancestry and blood quantum laws, which confer tribal status based on a person's amount of "Indian blood." (Indeed, as of 2019, the US Department of the Interior still issues Certificate of Degree of Indian Blood [CDIB] cards.)[63]

Race designation is more a matter of politics than science. As Professor Dorothy Roberts, an acclaimed legal scholar in race and gender at the University of Pennsylvania, suggests in her TED Talk, "The idea of innate racial differences in disease distracts from the social determinants that cause appalling racial gaps in health."[64] It seems race becomes biology, from the outside in.

> **Race designation is more a matter of politics than science.**

Another example of how cultural inequity becomes embodied is the "immigrant paradox." The contradiction goes like this: people who move to the US from places such as Mexico, Latin America, Asia, or Africa are likely to have *better* overall physical and mental health and lower infant mortality than later generations born in the US. Despite often not having much money, education, or health care to start, these immigrants experience an advantage that doesn't get passed down to subsequent generations. Full of hope, parents who leave their homeland behind believe their children will do better in the United States. Perhaps their own health is buoyed by their optimism and drive. Their children's health, however, is a different story.

> **It seems race becomes biology, from the outside in.**

It's unimaginable that a mother could go to such great effort to start over in a new place and then have children who fare worse in her new location, but that's exactly what happens. Though it seems highly counterintuitive, recent immigrants across ethnic groups fare better than first or second generations. The newly arrived have lower infant mortality, less violence, and lower rates of cancers, diabetes, and premature death than nonimmigrants or more established immigrants. A variety of studies across disciplines show that becoming an American is a risk for future generations living in the US, likely due to discrimination and other hidden factors that begin at birth and continue into adulthood.[65] Discrimination toward the US-born children of immigrants is ultimately more pervasive and longer-term than for their parents.[66]

Epidemiologists suggest that in the United States, our culture of inequality is likely the main reason why we rank last out of large peer OECD countries (Organization for Economic Cooperation and Development, aka club of rich nations) in life expectancy at birth despite spending comparatively 150 percent per person more.[67]

Despite the grim data, here is what I find encouraging.

Far outside hospitals and clinics, each one of us creates the culture in our day-to-day interactions and choices. We can make hidden factors explicit through discussion. Bias is a big hairy health problem that we all can do something about in our own circles of influence. The first step is to recognize that how I treat other people in my daily routines matters for my health, and how I let them treat me matters too.

> Our culture of inequality is likely the main reason Americans live shorter and less healthy lives despite spending far more on health care.

Sometimes we are on the receiving end of someone else's bias, and sometimes we dole it out ourselves. It is something we both give and get. With awareness and courage, we have the power to look bias in its Cyclops eye, whether it is in our workplaces, our schools, or a doctor's exam room. To address it also requires recognition that as humans, we mess up regularly, even if we consider ourselves "woke" to social differences.

Evidence suggests race is socially determined, which makes it tempting to act like we are colorblind. I remember my grandmother Tutu telling me at the dinner table that she did not "see color" as a way of saying human beings are all equal. Many Americans have adopted that approach with the best of intentions. But the risk is, we are blind to our own biases. It's like a drunk guy trying to grab car keys, shouting, "I'm fiiiiiiiiiiiine!" It's hard to see how your own judgment might be off. By not addressing differences directly, even if we think we are being polite, we can be doing more harm than good. Race is arbitrary, but it has too many real life-or-death consequences to ignore.

For those who don't face day-to-day discrimination, inequality may feel like something "out there" that *someone* should do *something* about, not a thing happening right in front of me that I play a direct role in multiple times a day. But it is, given the multidimensional nature of bias. In medicine, we need to both pay attention and have courageous conversations as individuals and as institutions. Instead of acting colorblind, we need to make a much more concerted effort to address how bias becomes a hidden factor in health. While coffee isn't nearly as life-or-death as the hospital, Starbucks took hidden stereotypes seriously when it temporarily closed eight thousand stores across the nation in 2018 so 175,000 employees could talk in small groups about implicit bias after a high profile racial bias incident at one of its cafés. It seems we all can treat each other with even more kindness.

It's not just what we say, but what we do. Our nonverbal communication is important too. For example, one study found no differences in what a doctor said to black or white patients discussing end-of-life care options, but what the doctor did was another thing entirely. With a black patient, the doctor was significantly less likely to stand beside the bed or touch the patient in a caring way as with white patients. Also, the doctor spent more time with his arms crossed, looking at the nurse or monitor. In other words, they showed less nonverbal compassion.[68]

I've often wondered what I might say if I were back in that situation with the department head who couldn't find "any qualified women" for the job. Perhaps I would mention the studies to him (he is a researcher, after all), or ask if the department has tried some of the software available now (see the box on page 124) to help diversify hiring. Or maybe I would suggest some organizations or individuals who could refer qualified candidates. If you've ever found yourself in a similar situation, you know that it's tricky. But the more we speak up with specifics on how to foster long-term change and inclusivity in the workplace, the better everyone's health will be.

The good news is, biologically, the human brain is hardwired for empathy. Like a secret trust fund, it is there for us to tap into if we remember the passcode. Neuroimaging shows that an area of the cerebral cortex known as the right supramarginal gyrus (rSMG) is crucial to empathy. It helps us put ourselves in someone else's shoes and avoid blatantly biased social judgments.[69] However, when we are rushed or making quick choices, like in the ER, our brain tends to bypass this process and just go with our gut impression. In other words, the stereotypes we hold, right or wrong, guide us to snap decisions. Neuroscience studies show people vary in their ability to suppress snap judgments not just from person to person but also compared to themselves. Data shows it is harder to overcome bias when we feel tired or stressed.[70] So this might be yet another good reason to put down our smartphones and go to bed.

Activities such as loving-kindness meditation help us tap into our empathy reserves and think more clearly when faced with a situation in which we may act rashly. The method as meditation teacher Jack Kornfield describes it is "to use words, images, and feelings to evoke a loving kindness and friendliness to oneself and others."[71] It often includes repeating phrases such as "May I be filled with loving kindness," "May I be joyful," and "May I be grateful for all I have." Once you've gotten to a good space with yourself, you can offer some loving kindness to others, even people you may not like. I find it kind of cracks me up, lightens the mood, and keeps me out of some trouble to say, "May *you* be filled with loving kindness, guy tailgating me."

Another option to reduce hidden bias is to swap out our go-to images, or heuristics, so we essentially reprogram our thinking for the inevitable quick decisions. Hundreds of studies based on the work of Harvard University psychologist Dr. Gordon Allport show that increased social interaction with diverse groups, especially when participating face-to-face in a shared activity, is one of the most effective ways to reduce bias and stigma.[72] Examples of this "Intergroup Contact Theory" include the Living-Learning Communities at the University of Michigan that Dr. Steele and his colleagues created.

At Columbia University's Vagelos College of Physicians and Surgeons, I worked on a program designed by Dr. Janis Cutler to have all first-year medical students visit a "living museum" founded by Dr. Janos Martin on the grounds of Creedmoor Psychiatric Center. The museum space features extraordinary artwork—paintings, drawings, sculptures, mosaics, and photography—created by people living with mental illness. The students visited the studio in small groups and the artists led tours, answering questions about their work and influences along the way. Beyond appreciating the imaginative and often vibrant art, the idea is to have medical students see the person behind the diagnosis. There is something so powerful about feeling accepted for who you are as a human being, beyond a label. In addition, the positive connection is good for our health too.

Or maybe implicit bias is a bad habit to be broken. This is the perspective of researchers in Madison, Wisconsin. A series of studies led by Dr. Patricia Devine shows that people who participate in the Madison "habit-breaking" interventions have dramatic reductions in implicit bias compared to controls, and that the effects persist months later.[73] For example, by just participating in a two-and-a-half-hour gender-bias-reducing workshop, STEM departments at a large public university increased female faculty hiring nearly 50 percent in the two years that followed compared to other STEM departments at the same university that did not take the workshop.[74] College students who took a seminar to reduce racial prejudice saw a dramatic drop in implicit bias scores compared to controls and, two months later, remained more aware of potential discrimination.[75] Interestingly, across studies, the people who had the greatest reduction were those who had the most concern about discrimination, so by reading this chapter, you are ahead of the game.

Fairness affects health profoundly, and its scope expands far beyond clinics and hospitals. This chapter begins to highlight the importance of equity in health and hopefully will kick-start discussions on how to help address it. Creating a culture of fairness where we can all thrive depends on your conversations and courage at dinner tables, grocery stores, coffee shops, cocktail parties, boardrooms, universities, preschools, and beyond. You never know when you'll be needed to speak up. In the next several chapters we'll see how the whole picture of our health requires recognition of the connections between mental processes (feelings, thoughts, and behavior), the physical body (cells, organs, and structures), and the hidden factors. We'll start by looking at the role of compassion in our environments.

EXPAND YOUR TOOL KIT
Practicing the Golden Rule

Discussing our differences peacefully takes tremendous courage. Ignoring differences between us (i.e., acting "colorblind") prevents us from fully being an ally for each other. If you feel you've been discriminated against, with whom or where might you safely discuss the situation? As we will talk about in chapter 10, there is power in groups and in sharing your story. The following are just a few ideas to start the conversation.

➤ To boost awareness of unconscious bias, consider taking the anonymous Implicit Association Test at https://implicit.harvard.edu. *Warning*: It may make you think twice about your near-and-dear beliefs.

➤ Volunteer to do an activity with people outside your usual social group. Participating face-to-face in a shared activity can make you see the world differently. Take your kids along. It is life-changing. If you have more time, consider a year of AmeriCorps, Teach For America, Senior Corps, or the Peace Corps. (See page 200 for my AmeriCorps story.)

➤ In the organizations you belong to, what safeguards can you put in place to promote fairness in hiring or promotion or salary practices? Frame it as a health issue. For example, innovative businesses are using software (e.g., Textio) to review job postings for hidden bias on both gender and ethnicity. This software screens for a "gender tone meter," a clever way to try to address implicit bias. (Companies like Johnson & Johnson have dramatically increased their hiring of women using such technology.)[76]

> Support state and national initiatives for pay equality and transparency, understanding that unequal pay is a hidden health tax for all of us. (If you work in health care, check out the Time's Up HealthCare Initiative.)

> Check out strategies from the Madison approach to "break the prejudice habit."[77] Consider an evidence-based workshop for your workplace.

> Tap into your own empathy reserves during challenging situations using techniques like loving-kindness meditation. (I used it this morning.) Consider taking an online or in-person guided session or class.

> If you are comfortable sharing your story, post to MicroAggressions.com or peruse the posts to build your own cultural sensitivity.

> If you are concerned bias may be playing a role in your diagnosis or medical care or that of a family member, ask the doctor, "What else could this be?" or "How else might his symptoms be treated?" If something feels off, please ask for a second opinion and listen to your intuition. Doctors are human too.

> Part of civil discourse is calling out double standards or blatant discrimination directly. Courage to navigate conflict and developing the skill set is a huge part of kindness. (See chapter 10.)

Chapter Eight

Environmental Influences:
The Power of Compassion

A very little key will open a very heavy door.
—CHARLES DICKENS

The psychiatric ER is the intensive care unit for wounds invisible to the naked eye. People often show up for what they need most: kindness and understanding. Those struggling the most with physical illness often share similarities in their backgrounds—mistreatment, discrimination, poverty, lack of healthy food, lack of stable housing, or social isolation. Noticeably absent is love—the kind that instills a sense of belonging and purpose.

That's why I felt surprised to see Chloe.

When Private popped up on our board of names, my ER colleague Dr. Reza Amighi asked if I could go see the patient. The designation is used as an extra precaution to conceal the identity of someone well known, which in a Manhattan hospital is fairly common. "Thirty-four-year-old woman. One prior suicide attempt. Came in this morning with a big overdose. Housekeeper found her down on the bathroom floor with a bunch of empty pill bottles. Empty bottle of gin, I think too. Labs are pending. She's already gotten charcoal." (Activated charcoal is a solution given in an attempt to try to reduce the absorption of a toxic substance in the gut and decrease fatalities.) Always a considerate clinician, Dr. Amighi said, "I have a hunch she'd prefer a female doctor."

I logged in to the computer to look over her history. I clicked on the Private tab and saw Chloe's famous last name appear. Her father was a chart-topping musician who was known for his upbeat sing-along melodies. Her younger sister, Samantha, was an award-winning actress. Chloe herself had had a successful modeling career as a young woman. In glossy magazine photos, their life seemed picture perfect, with glamorous parties, stylish clothes, high cheekbones, and big smiles. I now wondered what lay behind those smiles. I often think about the scene in *The Wizard of Oz* when Dorothy and her ragtag crew finally meet "The Great and Powerful Oz." After a big smoke-and-mirrors show, Toto yanks back a hidden curtain. There stands a frazzled, gray-haired man in a booth, frantically flipping a bunch of levers. Hoping to keep up the illusion, a booming voice says, "Pay no attention to the man behind the curtain." Working in mental health, my job is to peek behind that curtain. Sometimes I'd rather keep it closed.

Her sister, Samantha, stood by Chloe's bedside. Even though she had her hair in a topknot and wore jeans, she had a glamorous air about her. The unfettered confidence of someone accustomed to being watched. Chloe lay asleep on her cot, hooked up to a beeping monitor. Even while her pulse raced up to the 130s, she looked peaceful. Samantha said, "This feels so out of the blue. We were supposed to cohost a charity gala event tonight." She had gotten a call around 7:00 a.m. from the housekeeper, who said her sister was passed out on the bathroom floor. Thankfully, Samantha lived just one block away, and she ran straight over.

I looked at Chloe's platinum blond hair splayed across the pillow. The nasogastric tube taped to her nose lay dangling against her heart-shaped face. Samantha added, "I think she was saving up pills to take them. There were so many bottles." Chloe left no note. No explanation.

Samantha continued softly, "We got fitted for our gala gowns yesterday. She looked spectacular. Her dress is this velvet cobalt blue that matches her eyes. Our friend Alec designed it just for her. She didn't seem depressed. She seemed . . . fine." As her voice broke off, Samantha started sobbing, "How did I not see this coming again?" I squeezed her arm and stood quietly. Some risk factors are hard to see.

In 1945, after the end of World War II, the lights came back on in Great Britain. As life started to return to normal, people turned on house and streetlights again at night, no longer afraid of drawing unwanted attention from enemy forces. Around the holidays, festive lights illuminated town squares. People went back to going out in the evenings to see friends and attend parties.[1]

With more breathing room, researchers could think more broadly about the health of the people again. That's when epidemiologists clearly saw an unexplained problem: a surge in deaths from lung cancer. In the UK in 1922, 612 people died of the disease, whereas in 1947, 9,287 people died.[2] It was a staggering fifteen-fold increase in lung cancer, and public health and government officials hadn't a clue why. Great Britain had the highest incidence of lung cancer per capita, while rates skyrocketed around the world.

In the summer of 1947 in New York City, medical student Ernst Wynder sat in the Bellevue Hospital basement on a summer rotation. There he watched a pathologist do an autopsy on a man who had died of lung cancer. Ernst had traveled a long way to get to that moment. While he was a teenager, his family had fled Nazi Germany to avoid religious persecution. Then as a transplant to New Jersey, Ernst decided he wanted to dedicate his life to helping people. He applied to medical school and got into Washington University in St. Louis. He was in New York on a summer internship. That day, Ernst sat in the cool room and looked at the blackened lungs, thinking about the patient's widow.

Something the man's wife had said stuck out to Ernst: before the patient got sick, he had smoked two packs of cigarettes a day. It's hard to immediately remember that people haven't always known smoking was a huge risk factor for developing lung cancer, but the man's excessive smoking seemed rather a strange coincidence to Ernst.[3] He kept thinking about it and got the idea that maybe if he looked at other charts of patients who died of lung cancer, he'd find a pattern. Back in St. Louis, Ernst approached Dr. Evarts Graham, a pioneering thoracic surgeon who was renowned for his treatment of lung cancer patients. Dr. Graham was considered the Charles Lindbergh of surgery. Ernst, in a gutsy move for any medical student, asked the esteemed Dr. Graham if he could look through his patient charts to search for a link.[4] Dr. Graham initially declined, but with Ernst's persistence, he skeptically agreed.

Now, here is where we have to pause.

Reading this now, it is easy to see that the answer to the mystery is smoking. Of course, it's so obvious. But it wasn't at all. In 1948 about 80 percent of men smoked.[5] Doctors were no exception. Dr. Graham himself was a heavy smoker. And clouds of secondhand smoke surrounded those who didn't directly partake. Cigarettes in the 1940s were like cell phones today—ubiquitous. Instead of cigarette smoking, the leading hypothesis at the time was that the increased lung cancer rates were due to increased pollution from car exhaust, tar from new roads, factories, or coal fires. The cigarette idea seemed farfetched. In the 1930s, Scottish doctor Lennox Johnston was among the first to identify nicotine as addictive and suggest banning smoking, but he was way ahead of his time, and he was widely ridiculed.

In May 1950 the prestigious journal *JAMA* published Wynder and Graham's seminal study "Tobacco Smoking as a Possible Etiologic Factor in Bronchogenic Carcinoma: A Study of 684 Proven Cases."[6] The results, to modern eyes, seem ridiculously clear-cut. The researchers found the longer and heavier someone smoked, the greater their risk of lung cancer. An unmistakable health gradient. Only 2 percent of patients in their sample with lung cancer never smoked. The magnitude of the association between smoking and cancer was far too strong to reflect statistical bias alone.

In September 1950, like Wynder and Graham, two British researchers, Drs. Richard Doll and Austin Bradford Hill, published a preliminary report in the *British Medical Journal (BMJ)* that also found a strong link between smoking and carcinoma of the lung.[7] But at the time, the public, government agencies, and even many physicians ignored these seminal studies. Even Dr. Graham, one of the principal investigators, kept smoking. He eventually stopped in 1952.[8] By then, however, as Dr. Graham later wrote to Ernst Wynder, his coauthor, it was too late. In 1957 Dr. Graham died from lung cancer, the disease he'd dedicated his career as a surgeon to fighting.

Since so many doctors smoked and it was easy to locate them, Doll and Hill decided that they made a good group of subjects to study. To follow up on their initial findings, the team began to follow a cohort of forty thousand male and female doctors. The British Doctors Study, as it became known, ran for fifty years (1951–2001). Just several years into the study, an unmistakable pattern with heavy smokers emerged. In 1954 Doll and Hill published the first of two seminal papers in the *BMJ* that validated the causal link between smoking and lung cancer. It should have been major news. But only a few reporters at the time covered it, and those who did on TV actually smoked on camera during the announcement. The health minister of Britain at the time, Iain Macleod, did hold a press conference to announce the findings. Throughout the Q&A, he chain-smoked.[9]

Over time, findings from the British Doctors Study revealed the clear connection between smoking and cardiovascular disease, emphysema, and other types of cancer. So, too, did hundreds of other independent reports. You'd think with all that proof that medical practice and public perception would have changed dramatically. But it didn't. Ernst Wynder, Richard Doll, and Bradford Hill all endured decades of skepticism and even hostility over their results.[10] Over four decades later, in 1994, tobacco companies still testified in front of Congress that nicotine was not addictive and smoking did not cause cancer.

Sometimes the evidence of a clear risk factor from everyday environmental exposure can stare you in the face. But either through bias or blind spots, it is easily missed. Today evidence points to exposure to trauma as a similar blind spot. Like smoking, it's a health risk that has slid under the radar for decades. Environmental exposure to trauma, and particularly in childhood, proves another hidden factor in our health.

It may sound strange to talk about trauma as an environmental exposure in the same way we talk about cigarette smoke or chemical agents. But a toxin can be a chemical or a person or a situation. Traumatizing events, by definition, expose us to intense emotional distress, overwhelm our ability to cope, and leave us in fear of death. While adults can be exposed to trauma in a war zone or a serious accident or a sexual assault, as we will see, kids are particularly sensitive to the toxic stress of adverse childhood experiences (ACEs) with repercussions decades later.

In 1985 Dr. Vincent Felitti couldn't understand why a successful Kaiser Permanente obesity program in San Diego, California, had so many dropouts. It seemed when patients participated in the program, everyone lost weight. Some of the most severely overweight people lost over a hundred pounds. Then, right when momentum was on their side, nearly half stopped showing up. The weight would come rebounding back. Dr. Felitti and his colleagues were frustrated and perplexed. The participants had many advantages. All had health insurance through Kaiser. Most were middle-class, college-educated, and white.

Determined to figure out what was going on, Dr. Felitti started talking to patients. He asked everyone the same set of questions about their medical history. Then, by accident, he stumbled on an unexpected puzzle. During one of his many patient interviews, he fumbled his words, and instead of asking, "What age did you become sexually active?" he asked, "What weight were you when you became sexually active?" The woman responded, "Forty pounds." He recalled feeling confused. As the woman burst into tears, he understood what he'd asked.[11]

At the time, childhood sexual abuse was not something Dr. Felitti routinely asked patients about. He, like most doctors, considered it a rare occurrence. Plus, it felt embarrassing to bring it up when the person was there for what seemed like an entirely different reason. Yet after several more patients mentioned a history of traumatic instances, Dr. Felitti and his team decided to ask everyone more systematically. The results were shocking. Over half the patients with severe obesity had a history of childhood trauma. Dr. Felitti realized the odds of that association proving a coincidence were extremely low. In the 1980s, everyone thought weight was all about diet and exercise. I think about my mom's Jane Fonda VHS tapes now—everyone wanted to "feel the burn." So what in the world did trauma have to do with obesity? Dr. Felitti decided to present his initial findings at a medical conference for discussion.

> Over half the patients with severe obesity had a history of childhood trauma.

While his study would ultimately usher in a new era in human health, fellow physicians greeted his initial presentation with skepticism and even some guffaws.[12]

But one key person sat up and took notice. Dr. Robert Anda at the Centers for Disease Control (CDC) was intrigued by Dr. Felitti's work. He wanted to better understand the link between mental health and obesity.

Together, Drs. Felitti and Anda designed the large-scale Adverse Childhood Experiences (ACE) Study to verify the seemingly bizarre association. They sent out a survey to a sample of 13,494 adults with Kaiser insurance. The subjects were about 75 percent white, in their mid-fifties, and college-educated. Precisely 9,508 (71 percent) of people replied, which is a very good response rate for a survey study. The demographics of respondents were similar to nonrespondents.

Participants answered a series of questions about childhood exposure to adverse events, such as parental separation or divorce; emotional, physical, or sexual abuse; domestic violence; or exposure to a parent with a substance use problem or mental illness. Questions included, "Did a parent often or very often swear at, insult, or put you down?" "Was your mother (or stepmother) pushed, grabbed, slapped, or had something thrown at her?" and "Did a household member go to prison?" The number of yeses to ten key questions indicated the participant's ACE score. (If you want to know your score, check out online versions, such as https://acestoohigh.com/got-your-ace-score/.)

Drs. Felitti and Anda established that a history of childhood trauma is not rare, but a common occurrence. Their research found that half of all respondents had one or more ACEs, and a quarter had two or more. Adversity in childhood was twice as common in women as a diagnosis of breast cancer.[13] One in five people reported a specific type of adversity: a history of sexual abuse. As Dr. Felitti's initial study uncovered, a history of childhood trauma did significantly increase the odds of severe obesity.[14] While not every person who is obese has experienced a childhood trauma, the important takeaway is that adversity during childhood is a hidden risk factor for obesity as an adult.

And it wasn't just obesity.

The ACE Study, like the smoking studies, identified a clear dose-response, or what doctors call a stepwise graded pattern, not only to obesity but also to all the leading causes of death in adults. The greater the exposure, the bigger the effect. And as we know, this is exactly what causes epidemiologists to take notice. In other words, exposure to childhood trauma increased the risk of all causes of disease in the adult. This includes cancers, chronic obstructive pulmonary disease (COPD), heart disease, lung and liver diseases, and even sexually transmitted infections.[15] Compared to patients with no childhood trauma, patients with an ACE score of four or more also had a four-fold risk of alcoholism and a tenfold risk of using IV drugs.[16] Doctors typically talk about biological predispositions to addiction or even "addictive personalities," but it seems environmental exposure to trauma is a key risk factor.

As a young child, I remember my parents protecting me from my step-grandmother "acting funny." Visits to her home often ended abruptly once she got that gleam in her eye. As the years would pass, I'd see how she was absolutely lovely when she didn't have her gin and absolutely horrible with it. A totally different person disguised in the same body. Fragments of the past began to make sense, like the time she insisted I jump off the diving board into the deep end of the pool to get a ball even though I couldn't yet swim. Growing up, I wondered, what was wrong with her. Now I wonder, *What happened to her?*

Childhood trauma increased the risk of all causes of disease in the adult.

Numerous follow-up studies have confirmed that negative emotional experiences as a child create downstream physiological changes in the adult. For instance, a study that showed patients who had six or more ACEs got diagnosed with lung cancer on average thirteen years younger than those without ACEs.[17] This statistic in particular stood out to me, since lung cancer is what eventually killed my step-grandmother. While an increased risk of smoking plays a role, it doesn't adequately account for the findings. There is another physiological process at play. Study after study tells the same story: unaddressed ACEs shave years off someone's life.

At the heart of the health effect of trauma is toxic stress. *Toxic stress* crosses a threshold from a tolerable response to "severe, prolonged, or repetitive" physiological activation.[18] According to the Center for the Developing Child at Harvard, prolonged stress system activation for a child in the absence of a protective adult relationship is toxic to the body. While adults can experience adversity, too, such as PTSD in veterans, its impact is amplified on growing bodies. If left untreated, an exposure to trauma in childhood has long-lasting aftereffects that can change lives for the worse.

Childhood trauma is a critical missing piece of the health puzzle that most people keep hidden out of sight, stuffed under the couch cushions, because of the perceived taboo of talking about it. Given the far-reaching effects, you would think I learned about ACEs in medical training. Instead, I first stumbled across Dr. Felitti's work through a lawyer friend who was researching potential health effects after a family trauma. I felt a mix of relief and shock as I read the studies for myself. Relief for an explanation for the day-to-day clinical mysteries I saw in the hospital. I also felt shock, since I hadn't heard one word about ACEs in my decade of medical training from medical school through fellowship or in all the continuing medical education that followed. Perhaps someone did mention it, and it was so beyond my understanding of health that I didn't pay attention. In many ways, I'm like the doctors I scoffed at who were around during the time of the landmark smoking studies. While I was reading about the latest glitzy personalized medicine findings, I missed the big story that affects every other person I see.

Like Chloe.

Beneath Chloe's polished veneer lay decades-old trauma. As a child growing up in California, her younger brother, Sebastian, chased a ball into the street while he and Chloe played in the front yard. In the late afternoon sun, they never saw the sky blue Volkswagen bus turn the corner. Her parents told her that Sebastian's death wasn't her fault, but she never forgave herself. Even though she was only eight at the time, she felt responsible.

After her dad left, Chloe watched her actress mother carefully conceal her depression from the outside world. While her mom drank heavily and abused the pills a doctor gave her for her back pain, she always had an effervescent smile ready for the cameras. Chloe's glamorous mother had a parade of famous boyfriends, one of whom was a particularly charming actor on-screen, but was an off-camera sexual predator. Chloe was only twelve years old when he abused her for the first time. She felt so ashamed that she didn't say anything to her mom. Plus, Chloe was afraid of what he would do if she did tell. She'd often seen him push or hit her mom during heated arguments. That summer, Chloe tried to drown herself in the family pool. A gardener pulled her out and performed CPR. Her mom never took her to get medical help. Instead, perhaps out of fear, she privately berated Chloe for her actions. As the years passed, Chloe concealed her waves of pain and alcohol binges from Samantha. As the older sister (by three years), Chloe had seen herself as Sam's protector growing up. Only now the tables had turned.

From seeing Chloe's photo in a magazine, you'd never suspect she had an ACE score of seven. That's what's so sneaky about ACEs. Compared to someone without a history of childhood trauma, Chloe had over a thirtyfold increased risk for a suicide attempt as an adult. And she'd had a fifty-one-fold increased risk when she was a teen. Suicide risk goes beyond depression or substance use alone. An extensive follow-up study done by Drs. Anda and Felitti and colleagues, published in *JAMA* in 2001, showed that for every increase in ACE score, the risk of suicide attempts increased by 60 percent. The authors described how the link between ACEs and suicide risk is so pronounced and clear that rarely is such a robust association seen in epidemiology.[19] Perhaps aside from the smoking and lung cancer studies.

> The link between ACEs and suicide risk is so pronounced and clear that rarely is such a robust association seen in epidemiology.

The overdose wasn't out of the blue after all.

Great, you're probably thinking, *but now what? What do I do if I have a history of trauma or childhood adversity?*

So though there's a lesson in here for everyone, it's especially true of those with high ACE scores: to properly address the hidden factor of adversity or trauma, we need to look at how we can foster compassion for others and ourselves. Until someone invents time travel, we have to learn to navigate living with a history of adversity. It is tempting to move on and push it under the rug. It's what many of us, like Chloe, learn to do as kids out of fear and a desire for normalcy. The problem with that approach is that related symptoms can surface at unexpected times, blindsiding us or loved ones. Studies indicate that trauma suppression elevates the chronic stress response, and worsens PTSD, anxiety, and depression symptoms.[20]

> To properly address the hidden factor of adversity or trauma, we need to look at how we can foster compassion for others and ourselves.

The good news is that there is far more we could be doing.

It starts with self-care and self-compassion. Self-care is critical for healing. It is counterintuitive, but to be a better parent or spouse, make tending to your own emotional well-being, stress levels, and relationships a top priority. Pay attention to your own warning signs and patterns when you're going to lose it. Step away or distract yourself to cool off. Practice connecting with your child or partner before jumping in to correct behavior. Talk about behavior only after everyone has cooled off.

Healing also requires that we have compassion for ourselves. For adults, mindfulness techniques borrowed from holistic Eastern medicine traditions are helpful for boosting self-compassion. Like meditation, mindfulness training can help maintain focus on the present moment and improve positive thinking patterns. Evidence shows that cognitive reappraisal, or reframing a terrible situation, can help a person reduce her stress response and better cope when intense emotions emerge.[21] Therapies such as Dialectical Behavior Therapy (DBT)—created by Dr. Marsha Linehan, a researcher who has courageously spoken about her own experience with mental illness—helps participants develop these coping skills and reduce roller-coaster emotions through a process of radical acceptance.[22]

How we learn to live with an experience or loss that will never be okay evolves with time, and it can take years. Yet there is hope in the journey. Research shows there is some truth to the Rumi quote, "The wound is the place where the light enters you."[23] In other words, it turns out that adversity can be transformed into a positive force. The work of psychologists Richard Tedeschi and Lawrence Calhoun shows that adversity can empower people in significant ways such as seeing new life opportunities, forming increased connection and compassion with others, realizing one's own strength, and finding a deeper meaning in life.[24] Finding personal meaning in living with trauma is associated with less mental distress, better relationship satisfaction, and better physical health.[25] This phenomenon goes beyond resilience and is known as *post-traumatic growth*.

Interventions for growth don't have to cost a lot of money. For example, evidence shows that even writing about a painful experience from the past can improve immune functioning. And you don't need to produce a dissertation. Brief, focused writing seems to do the trick. In a classic 1988 study by James Pennebaker, Janice Kiecolt-Glaser, and Ronald Glaser, fifty undergraduates were asked to write about either a traumatic experience or an assigned everyday topic. Those who wrote about the traumatic experience were asked to write about the most traumatic and upsetting experiences of their entire life that they had maybe not talked about with others in detail. The instructions said the "important thing is that you write about your deepest thoughts and feelings." The writing lasted only about twenty minutes, four days in a row. Subjects were blinded to the reason for the study and researchers to the condition of the participants.

Then the researchers waited.

Six weeks later, the students who wrote about trauma reported a better mood, less subjective distress, and fewer visits to the student health center, and showed improvements on serum markers of immune functioning. Overall, their autonomic nervous systems seemed more chilled out.[26] Subsequent follow-up studies show benefits across age, gender, social class, culture, and even personality type in as little as fifteen minutes a day of writing for three days. Participants who form a narrative to make sense of how a negative experience has helped them grow as a person saw the most significant boosts in mental and physical health.[27] Also, these studies show this practice is helpful for stressful life events like a job loss, a cancer diagnosis, or the death of a loved one. Creative writing can serve a similar purpose and has been used as a tool to help children and adolescents process traumatic events.[28] It seems that expressive writing about traumatic experiences can serve as a form of low-cost preventive intervention for many people.

> Participants who form a narrative to make sense of how a negative experience has helped them grow as a person saw the most significant boosts in mental and physical health.

Overcoming trauma isn't something we must do alone. In fact, the steps we could be taking to address trauma have some surprising links to what we discussed earlier about Okinawans—and the importance of intimate bonds. Study after study shows the best way to buffer exposure to adverse childhood events, as well as other toxic stress exposures as an adult, is to foster relationships of understanding and support. Our relationships or social ties make a crucial difference to our mental health, and thus to our physical health. While we can't change the past, we can help immunize ourselves against negative effects in the present through empathy, compassion, and emotional connection. Our mirror neurons help explain why.

As human beings, we develop a timeless sense of self that doesn't age with the body. When I was seven or eight and my grandmother Tutu was well into her seventies, she told me one night that she felt the same inside as she had when she was my age. At the time I thought it sounded nuts, but now, many decades later, I understand. Even though the over 37 trillion cells of my body have swapped out and replaced themselves many times over, I'm still me.

To have a sense of self also requires us to have an understanding of "other." So when does our brain develop that skill? In the 1970s developmental psychologist Beulah Amsterdam placed eighty-eight babies from ages three months to two years in front of a mirror. Amsterdam also secretly put a smudge of rouge on each child's nose. She observed that a baby that was less than a year old seemed to think the fellow in the mirror was a silly playmate. The child made no move to wipe off the smudge. By the age of two, the majority of children displayed "mirror self-recognition" and touched their noses when they saw their reflection.[29]

Distinguishing between self and other is helpful for perspective taking, developing compassion, and keeping secrets. This skill is what psychologists call the "theory of mind." This developmental milestone, which begins around the age of four, helps us understand that we have different perspectives. This skill is tested by placing a yummy piece of chocolate in a Band-Aid box, showing the open box to a child, and then asking her what another person who comes into the room will think is inside the box. A child with a developed theory of mind, or perspective taking, will say "a Band-Aid," and a child without will say "chocolate." This skill can be taken a step further by taking a lovely gift box and hiding a plastic cockroach inside. Most three-year-olds can't pull off this practical joke, but most five-year-olds think it's hilarious.[30] Knowing that others may see the world differently than we do helps us develop our sense of humor.

It also helps us move from empathy to compassion and take things in stride. Unlike compassion, empathy is unfiltered. Empathy is feeling the pain of others acutely. It first develops in children, before the strong sense of "you" and "me" emerges. After my two-year-old son Zay tripped at the playground, he wasn't the only one who cried—his two uninjured best friends, Louis and Pearson, did as well. The work of psychologist Paul Bloom at Yale shows that babies can show empathy as early as three months.[31]

With typical brain development, one learns by about the age of five to identify when someone else is hurt or sad, but not break down with him. That recognition coupled with a sense of individual agency allows us to comfort our friend and get them the help they need. It's the difference between *empathy*, feeling what someone else is feeling, and *compassion*, recognizing someone else's emotional state and seeking to alleviate it. The distinction is not merely a semantic one. Imaging studies show different parts of the brain activate in these tasks.[32]

While humans have a sense of self and others for emotional connection, we are also connected with others neurologically, in part through brain cells called mirror neurons.[33] When you watch a friend reach for a mug of coffee, areas in your brain's motor cortex activate as if you are reaching for the mug too. This neural reflection allows us to intuitively understand the intention of others and helps us work cooperatively, by passing your friend the sugar, for instance. Mirror neurons enable us to copy other people's movements, such as when dancing. Interestingly, the more two people's actions are synced, the more cooperative they feel with each other.[34] (Perhaps this explains the psychological power of military drills marching in unison.) Other mirror neuron studies show similar copycat brain responses after seeing someone else smile, experience pain, or act violently. It is an astonishing ability of the human mind to mentally mimic the world around us and place ourselves in others' shoes.

That said, when we mentally mirror another person's experience, even though we feel it, we don't usually act it out. We can separate an action as not our own because other areas of the developed brain inhibit the activity associated with the thought. Researchers know this by studying disorders of inhibition such as Tourette's syndrome, a movement disorder that can cause physical and vocal tics. Studies show that if a part of the brain known as the supplementary motor area (SMA) is excited through transcranial magnetic stimulation (TMS), people without Tourette's syndrome will involuntarily copy others' actions as if they had the disorder. The SMA is one of the areas of the brain where researchers have found mirror neurons.[35] The reciprocity between others' actions and our own creates a strong sense of connection.

Resonating with someone else physiologically in an unfiltered way is helpful in supportive relationships. Perhaps this is one of the ways that talk therapy works. On the flip side, without a buffer or in a negative relationship, it could be overwhelming. And if prolonged, it can lead to burnout or toxic stress. It's the dark side of empathy. And it makes sense, then, why people who are more empathetic are also at greater risk of burnout.[36]

Thankfully, because compassion uses a different part of the brain than empathy, it can help us put another person's experience in perspective. Research shows that empathy is the gateway to compassion, and compassion is a higher-level mental skill we can harness for growth and healing. Perhaps counterintuitively, even if we are the one who has suffered the trauma, showing compassion for others and helping them put their trauma in perspective may help heal our own. Perhaps this is why ample evidence shows that forms of talk therapy such as support groups and cognitive behavioral therapy are helpful for healing. These groups are not just about venting, which studies show can make people feel worse, but helping people together practice skills to reframe experiences and discover personal growth.[37] Plus, they help us feel bonded to others and less alone.

The best part is that compassion breeds compassion. By showing compassion, we buffer each other's stress and help one another deal with adversity. Together, we reinforce each other's personal growth.

When I started psychiatry training in the early 2000s, much of the treatment for trauma focused on fixing what was wrong with the person. It felt so judgmental. After all, the downstream effects of trauma can create some tricky behaviors such as emotional deregulation and a short fuse.[38] A brain that's been exposed to trauma has a hyperactive fight-or-flight response. This is highly adaptive for survival in an unsafe situation. To act quickly, the primitive amygdala (sometimes called the "lizard brain") takes charge and bypasses the far more reasonable but slower cortex. Neuroimaging studies show less communication between the amygdala and the dorsolateral prefrontal cortex (DLPFC) and associated "executive" centers in patients with ACEs.[39] The problem is, an amped-up amygdala is a lousy manager of day-to-day emotions. It pulls out a machine gun for every fly.

Emotional deregulation is common with borderline personality disorder. In some samples, three out of four people who carry this diagnosis have a history of childhood trauma.[40] Childhood sexual abuse in particular is an important risk factor.[41] One of the most agitated patients I ever saw in the emergency room was diagnosed with borderline personality disorder. She was a beautiful young woman who had had a horrible childhood. The problem is that sometimes putting a label on a person can further stigmatize someone who already is suffering.[42]

Thankfully, a new positive paradigm has emerged. Known as trauma-informed care (TIC), it provides people with more understanding and support. The fundamental idea shifts from asking ourselves and others, "What is wrong with you?" to "What happened to you?" It is a much kinder approach. This fundamental mind-set change focuses on strengths and treats people who have experienced trauma with dignity. TIC provides opportunities for meaningful personal transformation.[43] And it doesn't just mean talk therapy—it could be expressing your emotional journey through painting, drawing, quilting, writing, poetry, sculptures, musical theater, or even yoga.

Trauma-informed response training is happening across the country with law enforcement and others in the criminal justice system. In the training, participants learn how to identify symptoms of trauma, such as hypervigilance, numbness, flashbacks, and physical symptoms (nausea, trembling, or anxiety).[44] The training is vital because trauma is a common environmental exposure for all of us (including law enforcement officers themselves), and signs show up in every type of setting, from medical clinics to schools to workplaces to jails. The more we recognize how common trauma and ACEs are in the people we meet, the more we can support each other and heal.

Chloe had a long history of trauma that led her to my care in the emergency room that day. She had carefully concealed her wounds from a young age, and despite being surrounded by people, she felt alone. It's like she was a three-pack-a-day smoker, and her doctor and sister didn't know. For a kid, it seems having at least one caring, stable adult who believes in you, gets you, and treats you with dignity can make a world of difference. If it's not a parent, it might be a teacher, a friend's parent, or a coach. Just someone who conveys that you matter. Caring for others is a superpower we all have. You may be that one person for someone else right now. Despite all her seeming advantages, as a child Chloe never had that support.

> **Caring for others is a superpower we all have.**

This makes me even more determined to help other Chloes get the best care possible. In the same way that doctors screen every patient for smoking, the evidence shows we need to find a way for doctors and clinics to screen every patient for the hidden factor of ACEs too. ACEs are an essential part of our medical history, given the relationship between the number of ACEs a person has and their risk of asthma, stroke, diabetes, heart disease, and heart attacks.[45] Trailblazing pediatricians like Dr. Nadine Burke Harris in Northern California are far ahead of the curve by screening for ACEs. Yet many adult physicians don't know that screening is easy: just a ten-question checklist that doesn't get into gritty details and just gives a simple number instead of complicated results.[46] This way doctors don't have to worry about opening Pandora's box in a ten-minute visit and retraumatizing a patient.

The clear relationship between exposure to adverse childhood experiences and adult health outcomes illustrates the profound link between the mind and the body. The reality is that most of us have not won the lottery of life and have hidden environmental stressors that put us at risk for disease. Understanding, compassion, and support through trauma-informed care can help alleviate the shame and open the door to post-traumatic growth. It can also help us feel less alone. On the one hand, we are individuals going about our day-to-day lives, and on the other, we share a fundamental connection as humans that we are just beginning to understand. As we will discuss in the next several chapters, our ability to connect and support each other is the true foundation of health. The essentials of health start with recognizing the role of the hidden factors on stress and their impact on physical and mental health.

EXPANDING YOUR TOOL KIT
Creating Healthy Environmental Influences

Take a moment to think about how you might boost compassion for yourself and others, especially if you have a history of trauma. What activities have helped you heal in the past? Here are a few ideas to get you started in your process of learning how to best navigate adversity.

Know your risk: check out the ACEs survey.

> If you are a clinician, please consider screening for ACEs routinely. If you are a patient, ask if that's a measure your doctor tracks and supports to minimize the impact of ACEs.

> Keep in mind that a history of trauma is very common. Every other person you pass on the street has at least one ACE. If you have ACEs, be aware that you have lots of company: almost nine out of ten people who screen positive for ACEs have more than one.

> If you have experienced trauma or a traumatic loss (such as the death of a loved one), consider joining a support group. You may also want to consider a trauma-focused writing workshop. Studies show that connecting with others with similar experiences accelerates the ability to find meaning after trauma.

> Prevention matters when it comes to stopping the cycle. Mind your own emotional well-being first. Walk away when you feel you're about to flip your lid.

> If you feel overwhelmed, please seek out care from your doctor or a mental health professional. We all need extra support from time to time. If you can, gather some names in your back pocket before a crisis strikes. When you seek help, ask about trauma-informed care (TIC).

ESSENTIALS OF HEALTH

Chapter Nine

The Mind-Body Link:
Individual Health

The difficulty lies, not in the new ideas,
but in escaping from the old ones.
—JOHN MAYNARD KEYNES

One February morning, while working in the ER, I got a call. On the other end of the phone, I heard muffled shouts and commotion. Dr. Colin Peters, the attending emergency room doctor, said, "Can you come soon? I have a Jane Doe here who's making a scene. She looks schizophrenic." He paused to say firmly, "Ma'am, please get back on your stretcher. I'll talk to you in a moment!" Back to me he said, "I think I'm going to need to sedate her, but I want you to see her first."

As an emergency room psychiatrist in a busy New York City hospital, this is a familiar request. It's not unusual to have someone, identity known or unknown, creating a ruckus. My job is to figure out why. I never know what waits for me on the other side of the call. Sometimes, when I'm lucky, I have a few moments to sip my coffee and look through the patient's electronic medical record first. After all, the reasons a person may act out of control are many, and the patient's medical history provides the most important clues. Does she have a prior diagnosis of mental illness? If so, could it help explain this new state of agitation? It's important to keep in mind people with severe mental illness develop other medical problems that can cause behavior changes too. Teasing apart medical and psychiatric diagnoses is my area of specialty.

That day, I didn't have time to waste, and there was no medical record to review. I ditched my coffee, stood up, and hustled to Area B. Each emergency room consultation starts with a familiar row of *click-clicks* as I use my ID to unlock a series of doors to get to my destination. The emergency department, lit with unforgiving fluorescent light, is a labyrinth of sections labeled A through E, ordered in part by how long a patient can safely wait for a doctor to examine them.

For the most part, the system works. While each patient is important, there are only so many doctors and nurses to go around. Area A has the trauma bay: broken bones, motor vehicle accidents, and stab wounds. Also heart attacks, strokes, and serious infections. Area B is for important medical issues that shouldn't kill someone in minutes if the triage nurses were correct in their sorting. Area B also has a holding area for patients undergoing evaluation for unexplained behavior changes. It's the wild west of the ER. Over the years, I've seen patients rip out parts of the ceiling, flip over stretchers, urinate on the floor, and dance naked. For this reason, several security guards are positioned at the opening of the bay to manage the unexpected.

As the double doors swung open, I heard shouting. An older woman, maybe in her sixties, with a mop of brown curls and dark skin stood at the nurses' station. Her hospital gown sat askew, leaving her back partially exposed. She slammed clenched fists on the Formica countertop. As I approached, she turned toward me, looking over my shoulder. Eyes wide, she shouted, "What kind of service is this? Where's the bus to the Poconos!" As a family member of another patient passed by, she tugged his arm and shouted, "Please help me!" As the startled man walked off, she began sobbing. A hospital security officer, who stood an imposing six feet four, gently coaxed the petite woman to her stretcher. Once on, she popped right off and tried to climb onto a nearby cot occupied by another patient. The officer again intervened. She stayed put momentarily, rocking back and forth and attempting to disrobe.

I found Dr. Peters, the attending physician. "I'm guessing that's who you want me to see?" I said. He smiled, briefly. I'd known him since I was a trainee. He was an efficient clinician, a skill well suited to the ER. "What do we know about her?" I asked. "Not a lot to go on," he said, shaking his head. "As far as we can tell, she's new to us." What he meant is that the patient had either not visited our hospital system before or wasn't found under the details provided. In America, hospitals don't share medical records, even in the same city. Given that she had no identification, staff listed her in the system as "Unknown, One," age "123."

That morning in the ER, our patient eventually said her name was Ana. When asked her birth date, she said, "Ana." When asked what medical problems she had, she shouted, "ANA!" From the ambulance report, I learned that on that icy morning at 5:03, EMS found her wandering the street in her bathrobe and slippers. A concerned citizen had called 911. When the ambulance crew approached her, she had started screaming obscenities. She had no identification on her. The report stated little except in scrawled handwriting AMS, meaning altered mental status, to describe her confusion. When we asked her more questions, she glanced away, whispering under her breath.

We had no context for her behavior other than what had transpired in the last several hours. As a doctor trying to help a patient, this feels a bit like starting a movie near the end and trying to figure out the entire plot. By the time I was called, Dr. Peter had done a lot of the work and there was nothing in her chart to go on. Her vitals were fine, the initial physical exam was unremarkable, and there was no clear evidence of infection. Her blood alcohol was negative, as was her urine drug screen. The more causes of her altered mental status we ruled out, the more Dr. Peters felt confident that she was mentally ill. If not for her screaming and not providing identification, Ana would have been sent home. Dr. Peters made up his mind: "She's psychotic. She probably just stopped taking her meds and decompensated." He was confident enough to opt against brain imaging.

In medicine, the feet tell a story.

When Ana calmed down enough to let me examine her, I removed her skid-free blue hospital slippers and found Valentino red toenails. The polish was perfect, unchipped, and not grown out a single millimeter. When psychiatric symptoms emerge, they are usually not sudden. There's usually a period of days to weeks beforehand where grooming goes out the window. This may mean not showering, allowing hair to grow matted, wearing dirty clothes—and it certainly means not tending to one's nails. That morning in the ER, Ana could barely understand or answer a question, but her feet looked like she'd just come from a pedicure. Besides, Ana's hair, while disheveled, looked recently trimmed, with no signs of gray roots. Either this woman, who couldn't tell me her birthday, had recently cared for herself, or someone else had.

The goal of medicine is that when someone gets sick, she gets the right care, in the right place, at the right time, every time. To get the proper care, she first needs the correct diagnosis. But studies show that doctors get things wrong. A lot. One to two patients out of ten are misdiagnosed. And one in ten patients die from a doctor error. Based on autopsy reports, diagnostic mistakes cause at least 40,000 to 80,000 US deaths per year in the US and cause far more harm and disability.[1] That is akin to around 80 to 160 jumbo jets crashing a year.

How do doctors get things so wrong?

The culprit isn't simply bad doctors. Diagnosis is as much art as science. With thousands of diseases and only a few hundred symptoms, it's not always easy to pinpoint the cause of any single health issue.[2] Well-intentioned doctors make blunders dealing with complex medical systems. Multiple mini mistakes over the course of a patient's diagnosis can lead to catastrophic results. The X-ray taken at the wrong angle, the spot missed by the radiologist, the message from the lab that wasn't sent over, the report not seen by the internist. Like *Murder on the Orient Express*, it's tricky to pin the blame on one person. Researchers estimate that because these incidents typically go unreported, odds are, all of us, at some point in our lives, have or will experience either a missed, wrong, or delayed diagnosis.[3]

Odds are, all of us, at some point in our lives, have or will experience either a missed, wrong, or delayed diagnosis.

But sometimes the reason things go wrong reflects a deeper problem. Sometimes, a misdiagnosis reflects a form of flawed thinking. It reveals an MD's and Western medicine's hidden assumptions. Sometimes, the problem reflects a training that's made medical and psychiatric diagnoses two separate buckets rather than a complex interrelated system. The risk of misdiagnosis skyrockets in cases with a mental health component.

Studies show that people living with severe mental illness receive lower-quality medical care and are at risk of dying 28.5 years earlier on average than people without these diagnoses.[4] These two facts may be connected. Too often, once a person has been put in the category of "mentally ill," doctors chalk every new symptom up to psychiatric illness. A physician may close his mind to the possibility of nonpsychiatric causes of symptoms. Which is somehow worse, since people with severe mental disorders have double or triple the risk of heart disease, lung problems, infections, diabetes, and stroke.[5]

I remember the story of Claudia, a sweet woman in her fifties with a long history of schizophrenia and chronic grandiose delusion that she was pregnant with George Clooney's baby. One night, she came to the ER short of breath. The ER physician who saw her initially told her she was anxious because of her worsening delusions and medically cleared her to go home. But before she left, the psychiatrist on hand ordered a chest X-ray, which revealed that Claudia had pneumonia. These cases happen all the time—even with good doctors. And it can mean disastrous medical outcomes for patients. Cancer left unchecked, GI tracts impacted, or infections untreated.

And in the category of "worst of both worlds," even mental illness itself can be misdiagnosed and mistaken as a cause for behavior when it's actually a symptom of another underlying illness. Part of the problem is that the possible causes of altered mental status (or delirium) are numerous and complex. Many of the ten thousand or so diagnosable medical problems can present with behavior changes or vague physical complaints that can appear psychiatric. The long list of potential causes for delirium includes cancers, falls, heart conditions, metabolic disorders, endocrine disease, autoimmune conditions, bowel diseases, vitamin deficiencies, accidental poisonings, and urinary tract infections. Besides, there are no confirmatory blood tests for mental illness, so it's that much harder to prove that a diagnosis like schizophrenia is wrong.

The initial workup for someone with behavior changes is thorough, but not exhaustive. And the average emergency room is not equipped to do more than a first pass at figuring out the underlying, often complex, cause. The goal is to order enough clinical tests to arrive at the correct diagnosis while avoiding the "million-dollar workup"—excessive diagnostic testing that may have no added benefit to the doctor's reasoning and may cause potential harm to the patient. This is where we were with Ana. Would the benefits of further testing outweigh the potential harms?

Still, after seeing her painted toes, I harbored fresh doubts about Ana's underlying diagnosis. I went in search of Dr. Peters. I found him typing a note on a computer at the nurses' station. I shared my concerns that there were some inconsistencies on Ana's exam, meaning it wasn't so clear that her diagnosis was mental illness. I thought we should consider some brain imaging. As I said this, I could see a parade of new patients getting wheeled in, and Dr. Peters looked tense. He stuck to his first hunch: "I think it's unnecessary radiation—and extra time and money. I'm admitting her to psychiatry." Since I was the consultant on the case, there was little I could do other than state my objections. Because of the long waiting list for hospital mental health beds and few open spaces, Ana would remain on her stretcher in the ER overnight.

As the day advanced, I got busy with other cases, but my mind kept returning to the mystery of those toes. With Ana, I asked myself again what I always do: *What am I missing?* I hunt for an overlooked diagnosis in the way I would want other people to search for me if I were incapacitated. Then, I got a call from the Area B nurse.

Ana had a visitor.

Back through the maze of doors, I returned to Ana's bedside and saw a woman in her mid-thirties, wearing a gray business suit, holding hands with a now peaceful Ana. I saw the resemblance even before Alexandra introduced herself as Ana's daughter. "I've been so worried," she said. Apparently, the person who called 911 was a concerned neighbor who tracked down Alexandra at the TV station where she was a morning news producer. But he didn't know to which area hospital the ambulance had taken her mother. To find her mom, Alexandra had called ERs all over the city asking for "Anastasia Washington," to no avail. After many dead ends, hang-ups, and long periods on hold, she finally learned that an unknown patient at our hospital matched her mom's description. Within the hour, she was standing at her mom's bedside holding a family photo.

Alexandra put down her mother's hand and pulled me aside. "I'm worried," she whispered. "My mom's very confused. When I arrived, she called me by my grandma's name." The last time Alexandra had seen her mom was three days earlier, and everything had seemed perfectly normal. Ana had picked up her grandson, Theo, from kindergarten, brought him to her place, and made him macaroni and cheese, like she did every Monday. She was a retired nurse and had lived alone since her husband, Alexandra's father, died four years ago. Alexandra said her mom had no prior history of mental illness or dementia, which, medically speaking, made a sudden diagnosis of that now highly unlikely. As far as drinking and drugs, Ana had an occasional glass of wine, which ruled out substance use as a likely culprit.

I asked if Ana had complained recently about not feeling well. "Maybe she said something about feeling a little under the weather for the past several days?" Alexandra said. "The last couple of weeks she's seemed worn out. But it's understandable—her sister in Florida died last month. They used to talk every day."

I felt my stomach drop.

A stressful life event, such as the death of a loved one, can predispose someone to infection. The stress response elevates cortisol in the weeks that follow and can impair immune functioning. What seemed like a vague viral syndrome to Alexandra might have morphed into something far more sinister. I excused myself, and I found Dr. Peters typing another note. "I think we need a neurology consult right away." With this new information, he picked up the phone. We still didn't know what Ana had, but we knew it was not schizophrenia.

There's an ongoing mind-body problem in Western medicine. Even though the mind is considered the by-product of the brain, psychiatry has historically been "carved out" from the rest of medicine. This occurs both in how insurance companies pay (or, rather, don't pay equally) for mental health care as a covered benefit, as well as physically separating clinics and hospitals for patients with mental illness from other medical settings. Separate is not equal when it comes to mental health care.

Because mental health is not well reimbursed compared to procedural specialties, many hospitals across America have reduced the number of psychiatric beds in favor of expanding more lucrative services such as cardiology or orthopedics. This means patients who come into the ER and need admission to psychiatry frequently get transferred elsewhere, including freestanding mental hospitals. At the freestanding hospitals, medical services are not as readily available, often closing the door on an additional diagnostic workup. The physical and financial structure of mental health care in America reinforces the mind-body division in medicine.[6]

> Separate is not equal when it comes to mental health care.

This artificial division between minds and bodies—between mental and physical health—in medicine explains how Ana almost got sent to the wrong place. It also explains why her correct diagnosis was almost missed. Happily, we caught our error with Ana. But here's the deeper tragedy of the mind-body dichotomy that's reinforced daily in our hospitals and our health-care system: What if the division itself is both harmful and false? What if instead of teasing apart medical and psychiatric diagnoses, we took a step back and looked at how fundamentally *connected* mind and body are? And then what if we used what we know about how the hidden factors affect both body and mind to more effectively address our individual and collective health?

Physical health, mental health, and the hidden factors are like the three legs of a stool that supports individual and collective health (see figure 4).

It's a simple idea and a simple image, but for me, it was revolutionary. After all, biomedicine and so much of my training focused almost entirely on the body alone. Seeing the connection between mental health and physical health also makes so much sense of all the stories we've talked about so far. Why do we miss so many of the hidden factors? Because if we don't acknowledge that mental health is related to

RELATIONSHIP BETWEEN PHYSICAL HEALTH, MENTAL HEALTH, AND HIDDEN FACTORS

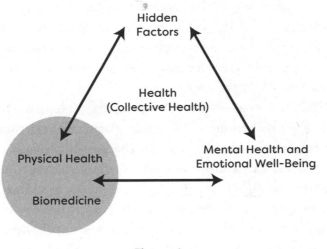

Figure 4

our physical health, we miss what's right in front of us. As we have seen throughout this book—from our relationships to our workplaces to our schools to our neighborhoods to how other people treat us to the adversity we face—what connects the hidden factors to poor health is often stress. And that stress, especially severe stress, as for Ana with the loss of her sister (and best friend), can dramatically affect our health.

So what is the mechanism that connects the mind to the cell? The key suspect in what links stress to disease is inflammation.[7] Incoming stress causes a cascade of changes in neuroimmune functioning that promotes systemic inflammation. Nonresolving inflammation is a significant driver of disease.[8] Pro-inflammatory cytokines released in chronic stress lead to general inflammatory states.[9] As we discussed in chapter 4, with Sylvie, pro-inflammatory cytokines released by the stress response give people "sick behaviors" like wanting to crawl into bed and rest. However, if the stress is ongoing or ignored, it leads to increased inflammation, which increases risk of all sorts of diseases, such as infection, type-2 diabetes, osteoporosis, heart attack, stroke, cancer, and mental illness. Prolonged stress is in itself an independent risk factor for poor health.[10]

Stress alters blood flow and healing in various body tissues. For instance, cuts heal several days faster for students on summer vacation (i.e., under less stress) than before exam time.[11] Similarly, cuts heal more quickly for couples in more supportive relationships versus more hostile ones.[12] But the healing time for cuts is just the tip of the iceberg in regard to stress's dramatic health effects.

In childhood, excessive or prolonged stress not buffered by a loving caregiver alters the architecture of the developing brain circuitry, as well as gene expression, through epigenetic changes.[13] This means potential health trouble decades down the road.[14] For example, one study looked at nine-year-old boys living in a stressful home environment versus children in a stable, nurturing setting. The stressful homes were replete with harsh parenting, less parental education, and persistent financial strain. The researchers found that children living with lots of environmental stress had telomeres 40 percent shorter than those who had more relaxed home lives.[15] (As you recall, shorter telomeres predict a shorter life and greater risk of developing a variety of diseases.) In addition, something important to consider is that the stress of exposure to frequent yelling alone may be as detrimental to a child's health as physical punishment.[16]

For a child, the stress of a prolonged separation from a parent puts that child at risk of diseases years later as an adult. Studies have found increased levels of inflammatory C-reactive protein in adults whose parents separated as children.[17] Meanwhile, oxytocin, or the "love hormone" released during cuddling with a loved one such as a parent, appears to double as an antineuroinflammatory.[18] It's as if Elizabeth Barrett Browning's love poem "How Do I Love Thee?" got translated into the carbon molecules of biochemistry. If love is nature's anti-inflammatory, it makes sense why its presence or absence has such a big impact on our health. And why cuddling the rabbits really did make a difference.

And here is where inflammation gets caught red-handed. The inflammatory process spans all bodily systems including the brain. And increasing studies indicate that inflammation appears to kick off many mental health conditions. We know this in part because there is evidence suggesting that psychiatric medications such as Prozac (for depression, anxiety, and obsessive compulsive disorder), lithium (for bipolar disorder), and Haldol (for psychosis) partially work because they are anti-inflammatory.[19]

When it comes to the relationship of mental and physical health, it often feels like a "Which came first, the chicken or the egg?" problem. For instance, inflammatory autoimmune disorders such as Crohn's disease and lupus notoriously flare with mental stress and in turn affect mood when poorly controlled. A patient named Maggie always knew a Crohn's flare was coming when she felt more tearful than usual. But if you step back and see the common underlying cause as inflammation, it makes more sense.

Given the mind-body connection, psychiatric symptoms are also sometimes an early harbinger of undetected disease.[20] Maureen, a corporate lawyer in her fifties with no prior history of mental illness, was admitted to the inpatient psychiatry service with two months of severe depressive symptoms, including apathy, hopelessness, insomnia, social isolation, and diminished appetite. The depression had come out of the blue, and Maureen hadn't responded to any of the typical treatments as an outpatient. Her doctor referred her for electroconvulsive therapy (ECT), which is one of the fastest and most effective ways to relieve depressive symptoms. After several treatments on the unit, she still was not responding. Sensing something else might be going on, we ordered abdominal imaging that revealed a tumor hiding out in the tail of her pancreas. The depression was an early warning sign of pancreatic cancer.

So we know that chronic stress leads to chronic inflammation and puts a person at risk of poor mental and physical health. And this stress arises from different areas of the hidden factors: relationships with family and friends, workplaces, schools, neighborhoods, or hassles we face in day-to-day life. We can think of stress as on a spectrum, where some stress is potentially positive on one side (like exercise or an alarm clock that gets us moving out the door in the morning). But at its opposite extreme it can veer into toxic stress.

Toxic stress, as we've seen with trauma, crosses a threshold from a tolerable response to severe, prolonged, or repetitive physiological activation.[21] Chronic activation of the body's stress-response system—the hypothalamic-pituitary-adrenal (HPA) axis—takes a cumulative toll. It can shorten life span if not alleviated. The result is what we saw with Randy. And Daisy. And Sylvie. And Ana.

With the medical history from Ana's daughter, Alexandra, we also ordered a stat MRI. Ana's symptoms without context appeared potentially psychiatric, but with the account provided by her daughter, there were glaring inconsistencies. She had no history of mental illness. Her symptoms came on suddenly and late in life. This unusual presentation, coupled with the fact that she was recently ill and had a significant social stressor, made an underlying infection far more likely. Fever, the usual red flag for infection, is less common in older people with inflammation of the brain's cerebral cortex.

Ana's MRI showed temporal lobe abnormalities consistent with herpes simplex encephalitis (HSE), a type of encephalitis more common in people over the age of fifty. A lumbar puncture (spinal tap) confirmed the diagnosis. We didn't do it sooner because spinal taps are invasive and uncomfortable for patients, and carry some risk of headaches, bleeding, or worse. In medicine, you have to have a good reason for doing a test and the potential benefits must outweigh the risks. Plus, on arrival, Ana had no headache or neck stiffness. The problem is that HSE can present with vague symptoms, and if left untreated, three out of four infected people die. For the one out of four who do manage to survive untreated, significant neurological impairments are common.[22] Patients like Ana who get the antiviral medication acyclovir early have the best shot at recovery.

The neurology service admitted Ana. With intravenous antiviral treatment, she improved. Ana became more like herself. By the time she was ready to return home several weeks later, she was very weak, but thinking more clearly and excited to see her grandson again. I ran into Ana as her daughter was helping to wheel her out of the hospital. I stopped them to say goodbye. Ana looked at me and asked, "Do I know you?" She had no recollection of the first week of her hospitalization. When Alexandra told her I was her doctor in the emergency room, Ana gave me a long, intense stare. After a lengthy pause, she broke out in a broad smile and squeezed my arm. I paused to think how differently her story might have ended.

Missing the link between mental and physical health is too common and serious a problem to ignore. Not only does the estrangement contribute to missed diagnoses, but it reinforces the stigmatization of psychiatric disorders by patients, families, and the general public. Diagnoses of the brain seen by neurologists seem like impersonal conditions that happen to someone, i.e., "Andy developed Parkinson's" or "Meryl has Alzheimer's disease." You don't hear, "Andy is Parkinson's" or "Meryl is Alzheimer's." Whereas diagnoses about the mind diagnosed by psychiatrists can feel like cruel judgments about character or identity, i.e., "Lou is schizophrenic" or "Jack is autistic." While it's more accurate to say, "Lou is living with schizophrenia" or "Jack has autism," the former is still common lingo.

The language used to describe mental conditions makes it easy to lose sight of the person living with the illness. The stigma can also cause people to feel apprehensive about seeing a mental health professional. I remember the first time I was called to the surgery floor to evaluate a patient for depression during my psychiatry training. I felt flustered when the patient's brother greeted me at the door in a huff and told me his sister didn't "need" to see a psychiatrist. He was upset with the surgery team for calling me. Somehow, I don't think dermatologists get that reception. I've now come to understand that navigating and reducing stigma for people experiencing mental distress is part of my role. It's an opportunity to engage families and increase awareness about the interplay between mental and physical health that is at the heart of this book. After all, mental anguish is widespread in the hospital: studies estimate that one in four people admitted to the general hospital have psychiatric symptoms.[23]

While Western medicine has been slow to recognize the mind-body connection, Eastern medicine traditions have always stressed its importance. In many Eastern practices, illness is thought to stem from an energy imbalance. A life force is considered part of the physical health. In Indian medicine and Ayurvedic healing traditions, *prana* is the term that describes universal cosmic energy. In Chinese traditions, this "vital force" is called chi or qi. Since around 500 BC, chi has been central to the practice of traditional Chinese medicine (TCM). The idea is that a human being and her surroundings contain energy that must be in balance for good health. A person is continually exchanging energy with her environment through her experiences. In Western medicine, with its singular focus on the physical body, this viewpoint has been mostly dismissed as "woo-woo."

As a medical student, I attended an optional seminar about TCM. I approached the talk with skepticism. I was intrigued but unconvinced. The practitioner discussed the importance of adjusting energy imbalances in the liver for ill patients. At the time, in the early 2000s, I thought this sounded outlandish. After all, I had no framework to unite my Western medicine model of human physiology with Eastern medicine's long-standing theory and practice.

But here's where things get exciting.

There are increasing rigorous scientific studies showing that exercises that bring the mind and body into alignment, such as synchronizing the breath and the heart rate in meditation, improve immune function and reduce the risk of disease and death. Compelling research shows that changing one's energy flow, or what the West might term reducing stress and increasing compassion, positively impacts tissues at a microscopic level throughout the body.[24] We now understand that an important marker for inflammation in the body, C-reactive protein, is produced by the liver in response to stress.[25] Yes, the liver. What sounded like hocus-pocus to Western doctors learning about Eastern traditions may on a microscopic level reflect the neuroimmune system at play. Because we did not understand it, we dismissed it. In Western medicine, we're just now embarking on the exciting new era of understanding the bidirectional communication between the nervous system and the immune system via autonomic and endocrine functioning.

Recognizing how much of our ill health can be traced back to the mind-body connection, stress, and the stress of the hidden factors illustrates a whole host of new paths we can take to better health. Many of these routes are free and preventive rather than expensive, after-the-fact treatments. Bolstering emotional well-being can help offset stress during challenging times, like when facing a personal crisis or illness. Actions that buffer stress are well within our grasp.

Now, I know I promised you this wouldn't be just another one of those self-help books with the usual directives: "Eat better, sleep more, work out!" And we'll get to the bigger picture of collective health soon. But I'd be remiss if I didn't suggest some actions you can take as an individual to boost your health. Knowing what we now know about the crucial importance of mind to body, it's impossible to ignore that our everyday acts to cultivate a healthy mind matter.

We can start by examining the possibility of a mind-body link in our own pains and ills. When new mental or physical symptoms arise, we can check in with ourselves as a first step. For example, when you have a new headache or back pain or belly pain or leg pain, take a moment to slow down and check in with how you are feeling in your body otherwise and what's going on in your life. Symptoms such as pain are a red flag for an underlying problem. And that problem may have to do with our mental health. We can ask ourselves, "Do I feel tense from stress? If so, where do I feel it in my body?" "Did I miss a good night's sleep or skip a workout?" "Did I indulge in unhealthy foods I wouldn't normally have eaten because of stress?" If so, what steps can you take to get back on track and introduce some relaxation? While, certainly, please do go see a doctor to check out symptoms that persist, you can do a first pass by considering your own mental state in relation to your physical health and making adjustments to see if it helps.

Like Ana, if you face an acute, intense stressor that knocks you off your feet, do what you can (recognizing that it's not easy in the moment) to take steps to buffer that stress immediately so little problems don't become big problems. Here is something I can suggest from experience having a family member in the intensive care unit. In the midst of a crisis, please take mini self-care breaks (i.e., catch a nap, take a brief walk, call a friend, or do whatever works best for you to mentally switch gears). Please ask for help from others so that you don't get too run-down. You'll be in much better shape to deal with what may come.

Another key way to buffer your health reserves is to take steps to reduce your baseline levels of negative stress. The idea is to get into the best mental shape possible so that when an acute stressor rocks your world, you'll be better able to stay balanced. Aside from getting regular sleep (seven or more hours a night) and exercise (see other books on ideas about this one), some other ways to reduce personal stress include meeting up with a friend for coffee (chapter 3), attending a regular support group (chapter 10), and journaling (chapter 5).

We can also build resilience through meditation and mindfulness. Taking a brief meditation break can help turn around a stressful day. Numerous studies have shown that people who meditate have significantly lower levels of stress hormones compared to non-meditators. Meditation also increases brain plasticity and help slow disease progression. For example, a five-year study followed high-risk black men and women with known heart disease. With regular transcendental meditation for twenty minutes twice a day (where participants focus on repeating a single mantra with their eyes closed), the study found a 48 percent reduction in the risk of heart attack, stroke, or other causes of death compared to people in a health education group.[26]

Meditation can help us recover faster from the slings and arrows of a challenging life. Research done by Professor Richard Davidson and his colleagues at the University of Wisconsin-Madison shows that long-term meditators, such as Buddhist monks, have brain reserves of resilience to tap into during difficult times.[27] The good news is that we don't have to shave our heads and take a vow of silence. Neuroimaging studies show increased activation of regions of the brain involved in altruism and emotional regulation after practicing loving-kindness and compassion meditation for thirty minutes a day for two weeks.[28]

Mindfulness habits can be cultivated practically anywhere, anytime. Some ideas to get you started: Take a walk without your headphones (or a drive with the radio off) and just pay attention to what you see around you. After dinner, my kids and I often enjoy walks around our city block where we just point out things we see. A variation is to stop and notice three things that are good right now. For instance, the way the sunlight hits the back of the leaves, the feel of the wind on your cheek, or how the ground feels so solid under your feet. You can also practice mindfulness while doing chores. Try it out while washing the dishes, paying attention to the rushing warm water, the soapy bubbles, the weight of the glass in your hand, the squeak of the plate. You get the idea. If your mind wanders off, wiggle your toes to bring your attention back to the present. Try to "Be here now."

In addition, we can practice gratitude, which has been shown to boost mood and reduce stress.[29] Consider the amazing people who have believed in you and helped you get where you are in life. (Thanks, Dad!) Take a moment to write a letter to someone, telling that person what he or she has meant to you. Practice gratitude for what you already have, and let the rest go. You don't need it anyway. Think about your spiritual teachers, who challenge you to become a better human being. They're not always formally trained. Spiritual teachers come in all shapes and sizes (my three kids are mine). Offer them gratitude. In addition, you can practice a random act of kindness to make someone's day and remind others of the goodness that exists. Buy someone a cup of coffee, let someone who seems in a rush go in front of you in line, take colorful flowers to a friend, etc. It will fill you with gratitude, too, and offset some of the sadness in the world.

Relatedly, cultivate a sense of awe. Nature helps remind us of our great interconnection and place in the universe. Plus, as we know from chapter 6, it boosts immune functioning. Consider going on a hike, run, or bike ride (don't forget the helmet), or visit a nearby body of water, check out the beauty of the ripples or waves, and enjoy the view. Look up at the constellations on a clear night and search for Orion or the Big Dipper. Spend time with a child or a pet and just marvel at how he navigates the world. Take a deep breath, relax, and smile at the incredible mystery of it all.

Have some old-fashioned fun to burn off stress. A few ideas to get you started: Take your own childhood delight in seeing a rainbow, or gently poking a roly-poly bug, or jumping in a rain puddle. Do something you used to love as a kid: doodle, play checkers, build with LEGOs, or throw a ball against a wall. Dress up for Halloween. For me, I get endless joy out of Skee-Ball or an afternoon at an amusement park. Grab a friend and go out dancing (which boosts fun and which studies show helps people live longer).[30] Do things that work for you and that you enjoy to lighten up and de-stress.

You may have noticed that many of these suggestions have in common a kind of positive thinking about the world and our place in it. That's no accident. Here is the remarkable thing, and what I wish I knew decades ago: there is evidence that stress about stress is a self-fulfilling prophecy. You are not a passive participant in the world. We are constantly appraising a situation and determining how to respond. Our amazing brains help us decide in a nanosecond if we need to run, freeze, or keep sipping our coffee. An exciting area of research shows that a person's perception of a stressful event as a threat (negative) or challenge (positive) may influence the body's reaction to it. In one of Mother Nature's bizarre practical jokes, it seems the more a person labels a situation as harmful or stressful, the more toxic it becomes.

> **There is evidence that stress about stress is a self-fulfilling prophecy.**

Several mind-bending studies indicate that high stress, plus the *fear* of stress, is an explosive combination. Researcher Dr. Elissa Epel studied the biological effects of stress on moms caring for chronically ill children. She designed a study to look at cellular aging among women with the highest levels of *perceived* stress compared to low-stress women. Her team recruited fifty-eight women, mostly in their late thirties, who had no known chronic medical conditions (i.e., they were healthy). The results were shocking: the women with the highest levels of *perceived* chronic stress had life span markers shorter on average by a decade compared with the low-stress women. In other words, the moms who reportedly felt most stressed out had biological life span markers shrunken to the length of someone ten years older.[31] Their DNA had fast-forwarded through years of potential good health.

It seems that how we perceive stress matters much more than the literal experience of stress. For example, one research group used data from the large National Health Interview Survey, focusing on people who reported a large amount of stress *and* who were chronically worried that stress hurt their health. (About four in ten Americans report losing sleep over stress.) The individuals who worried about the effects of stress had a 43 percent increased risk of premature death compared with those who experienced a lot of stress but did not perceive its effects as negative. Weirdly enough, the people with self-reported high stress and low fear of stress had the least risk of death. I guess some people love a challenge.

Further research suggests that 20,231 people die each year of stress plus the fear of stress, which would make it the thirteenth leading cause of death in the US. Stanford University psychologist and stress researcher Dr. Kelly McGonigal points out fear of stress may kill more people than skin cancer, HIV/AIDS, or homicide.[32] In addition, a large study that followed participants for eighteen years found that those who reported at baseline that stress affected their health "a lot or extremely" had over twice the risk of a heart attack compared with those who reported no effect of stress on their health.[33] It seems that stress is like a monster under the bed. If you worry about him, he's a nightmare. But he doesn't cause trouble if you don't believe in him, or he might even become a friend if you offer him a cookie.

Our ability to reframe adversity in a positive light, as discussed in chapter 8, is an important component of stress relief. While data suggests that objective stress has an effect regardless of how the people involved may feel—for example, in the Canadian ice storm studies, the number of days without electricity predicted the epigenetic changes in the babies, regardless of the mother's subjective stress level—a person's positive interpretation unquestionably buffers stress's toxicity. Let's face it. Stuff flies at us from every angle in life, from our family obligations to our work to the headlines in the newspapers. But like Wonder Woman's golden cuffs, a positive stance deflects stress and makes us feel more warriorlike in the process. (If only we could get our hands on a Lasso of Truth too.)

In Western medicine, our artificial separation of the mind and body interferes with our ability to see the bigger picture of health and address related hidden factors. Thankfully, Ana had a happy ending, but for every Ana there are jumbo jets filled with other patients whose diagnoses we missed. The reality is that the mind and body are physiologically linked and impacted by the hidden factors in ways we are just beginning to understand. We can use our understanding of how stress impacts our mental and physical functioning to boost our health. This model evokes the 1948 constitution of the World Health Organization (WHO), which defines health as "a state of complete physical, mental, and social well-being and not merely the absence of disease or infirmity."[34]

In the mid-2000s, the WHO furthered this call along with physician and public health leaders and health policymakers by launching a global campaign to educate people that "there is no health without mental health."[35] It highlights the substantial interaction between mental and physical symptoms and the enormous toll of untreated psychiatric conditions on physical health.[36] As we will discuss in the next chapter, for this movement to succeed, it needs you. We can all boost our collective health by addressing our hidden factors together.

Chapter Ten

All of Us (Trust):
Collective Health

The greatness of humanity is not in being
human, but in being humane.
—MAHATMA GANDHI

The year was 1978. In the midst of the Cold War, US senator Ted Kennedy found himself on a flight to Alma-Ata in the stunning snow-capped Trans-Ili Alatau mountains in the former USSR, what is now Kazakhstan. The World Health Organization (WHO) had invited Kennedy and leaders from around the world to cross the political divide and discuss an urgent matter in an unprecedented gathering. Over six days in September, the International Conference on Primary Health Care met at the imposing Lenin Convention Center in a "spirit of partnership and service."[1] Despite the looming threat of nuclear war, these leaders put aside their political differences to focus on the world's shared humanity.[2]

That the brother of a slain president and slain attorney general participated conveyed symbolic significance. The assassinations of Ted Kennedy's brothers resulted in not just trauma for the Kennedy family—deep distress that the senator's son Patrick later said his father suffered mostly in silence—but in a collective trauma for America.[3] The Alma-Ata Declaration was intended to address similar assaults on both personal and collective mental health. For the first time, a group of governments came together to say that health wasn't just about sickness or disease. Any definition of health, the leaders declared, must include mental health—and our overall social well-being.

But like this book, the Alma-Ata leaders weren't satisfied with just redefining health. They wanted a road map. They knew health occurs in a social context. If the roots of poor health rest in our social environment, then the solution to improving health does too. They asked, what if we all possess a "right and duty" to participate in health care? What if individuals, not just professionals, could provide preventive care for their fellow citizens? And with the radical idea that we could all help one another to better health, groundbreaking global steps to collective health were taken.

As we've traveled through the rings of the hidden factors, we've seen how our positive connections to one another start at home and in our neighborhoods. When a little girl feels physically and psychologically safe in her immediate environment, she's at ease. Her brain is more playful and creative. In her day-to-day life, she endures less negative stress, which means lower cortisol levels and less inflammation—putting her at reduced risk of developing diseases as she grows. When illnesses do occur, she copes better. Feeling safe is a key component of health.

But the positive benefits of good social connections don't stop with one child. What happens at the individual level—a person's emotional well-being and worth—can have exponential effects. A sense of warmth and support lifts a child's spirits. Feeling liked and valued, she's more willing to speak up and engage in school, in friendships, and in her community. She looks out for others and trusts that they look out for her. Eventually, as she grows, she nurtures and fosters trust in her own child. And it's not just her daughter who benefits. It's everyone. Because the secure child, now a secure woman, gives back the support and trust she was given. She'll help others feel safe, not just at home but in her workplace and her community.

That may sound like a nice parable, but it's actually an essential part of a thriving society. What we're discussing, and the thrust of the Alma-Ata Declaration, goes beyond the individual ("me") or community ("us").

It is a two-way dynamic partnership between an individual and her community that forms a sense of belonging, protection, and purpose. The network formed by our bonds to each other creates a safety net of collective health. While it starts in your home and mine, it has positive outcomes for all of us.

Collective health is akin to what Dr. Martin Luther King Jr. termed a "Beloved Community." With understanding and goodwill, all people can enjoy emotional well-being and the peace it brings, and share the earth's riches. In a Beloved Community, Dr. King wrote, "Poverty, hunger, and homelessness are not tolerated because international standards of human decency will not allow it." It's the responsibility of all of us to ensure that everyone has enough. The Beloved Community is the kind of place where "people are other-centered, not self-centered," where a man would go out of his way to help a stranger and two people with opposing viewpoints could become friends.[4] Dr. King believed this was realistic if a critical mass of people commit to resolving conflicts peacefully. So while Dr. King's vision remains unfulfilled, it is still attainable if the majority of us pledge to become active members. It starts one person at a time.

The Alma-Ata Declaration offered a glimmer of the Beloved Community about which Dr. King dreamed. Back in 1978, when the world seemed to be splitting apart at the seams, the participants in the conference knew that better health for everyone required collective action far outside hospitals and clinics. To realize the goal of the Alma-Ata Declaration, every citizen (that's you and me) must recognize her leadership role in community health. The gathering called for immediate action by "all governments, all health and development workers, and the world community to protect and promote the health of all the people of the world."[5] In short, the group devised a blueprint for collective health.

Just across the border from Alma-Ata in neighboring China, a developing nation at the time, the "barefoot doctors" program exemplified this new vision of health. This program illustrated that better health didn't require more dollars, just more innovative models. Barefoot doctors pioneered "task shifting." Rather than requiring that ultra-trained medical professionals provide all medical care, some of the responsibility shifted to community workers. In Western medicine, healing is concentrated in the hands of physicians at clinics and hospitals. But China's challenging population distribution necessitated a different approach.

In China in the 1950s most physicians lived in cities, while the majority of the country's population lived in the countryside. To meet their health needs, the government recruited local peasant farmers to take courses in primary medical care and first aid.[6] Classes focused on health for women and children. Participants learned about immunizations and hygiene, such as hand washing. A million barefoot doctors worked in the fields alongside their patients. Among other successes, the program significantly reduced the incidence of the freshwater parasitic infection transmitted mainly by snail larvae known as "big belly," or schistosomiasis, the second most common parasitic disease in the world behind malaria. Field studies showed overall a reported 10 million initial cases in China were reduced to 2.4 million.[7] One barefoot doctor at a time protected the same number of people from complications of schistosomiasis as the populations of Chicago, Houston, San Diego, and Phoenix combined.[8]

The barefoot doctors program was an outrageous low-cost success that provided immediate help where it was needed and could serve as a model for improving care around the world. It could even serve as a model in parts of the world where access to care is severely limited. And the participants at the Alma-Ata conference knew it. [9]

But here I am writing this over forty years after that unique summit in Kazakhstan, and I suspect that, unless you've studied public health, you've probably never heard of the Alma-Ata Declaration or the barefoot doctors program. Even as a physician, I hadn't. The declaration was a major milestone of global health that was then set adrift like a note corked in a bottle waiting to wash ashore. So with this bright vision in mind, how do we still get there? What tools do we need to build the Beloved Community and boost our collective health?

The principles of Alma-Ata and programs like barefoot doctors, pioneered in China when it was still a developing nation, can easily work hand-in-hand with today's world of Westernized medicine. But it does require a mind shift. Currently healing remains concentrated in the hands of physicians. If we truly want to improve health, we need to think outside the hospital. Interventions that shift responsibility from a handful of professionals to numerous trained community members are an exciting possibility, especially in cases where needs far exceed existing medical resources. Some task-shifting programs, many still in pilot phase, are already seeing amazing results.

Take maternity care. For eight hundred women around the world, pregnancy transforms into a death sentence every day.[10] Many women lack essential basic monitoring both before and after childbirth. Without proper pregnancy care, treatable conditions worsen and can lead to fatalities; globally, a mother dies every two minutes from complications related to pregnancy and childbirth. In the US, we lose two women every day in childbirth and 140 more come close to death.[11] (To get a glimpse of some of the challenges to giving birth in the US, check out the series "Giving Birth in America" available at https://everymothercounts.org/films/.) The most tragic part is that the majority of maternal deaths are preventable.[12]

Every Mother Counts aims to make pregnancy and childbirth safer for every mother, everywhere. The organization was started by human rights campaigner and beautiful human being Christy Turlington Burns. After she experienced a serious complication after the birth of her daughter, she decided to pursue a master's degree in public health and use her knowledge and platform to help save moms (and families). After all, women who die often leave behind devastated children, partners, and friends. The organization helps support respectful maternal care led by people in the communities where change is needed most.

Many women around the world lack access to skilled care during pregnancy, delivery, and postpartum. Clinics are often simply too far, underfunded, understaffed, and/or undersupplied. To bridge the gap, Every Mother Counts supports programs in underserved communities to help train midwives, nurses, traditional birth attendants, and community health workers to safely perform many of the tasks currently done by too few doctors. The aim is to identify, refer, and treat complications in order to curb preventable deaths and health conditions, in part, by training skilled birth attendants where they are most needed.

The results show midwives, doulas, and other birth workers dramatically improve maternal health outcomes. A 2017 Cochrane review found that the continuous support of women in labor, such as that provided by traditional birth attendants and doulas, shortens labor, increases natural vaginal deliveries, improves APGAR scores, reduces the use of pain medications and C-sections.[13] Plus, it's just so humanizing to have someone cheering you on in childbirth. In westernized medicine, to have someone support a woman throughout labor is rare, even though there are no adverse effects of this relatively low-cost intervention. The midwifery model of care, which is endorsed by the WHO, looks at the mother as a whole person and treats her with a level of compassion and kindness that is increasingly shown to improve health outcomes.[14] Plus because midwives and traditional birth attendants often come from the communities they serve, they are known, trusted, and provide culturally competent care.

If more supportive care is task-shifted from hospitals and clinics to the communities where people live, more health workers could be trained, addressing provider shortages at a lower cost, and hospital and clinic resources would be available for situations where they are most needed. In other words, more moms, children, and families could thrive. For example, a remarkable study published in *JAMA* in 1997 described the incredible results of a simple program of prenatal and early childhood home visits in a semirural community in the southern tier of New York State. The moms were 90 percent white and about half were unmarried or younger than nineteen. Compared to a control group that had the usual well-child clinic visits, the moms who got regular home-based prenatal care had better health and were less likely to use alcohol, tobacco, and other drugs. Rates of childhood abuse and neglect decreased too.[15]

Perhaps the most amazing part? The community home visits significantly reduced criminal behavior in the women's offspring fifteen years later. The kids were far less likely to run away, be arrested, be convicted of a crime, or violate probation.[16] Follow-up studies make the evidence crystal clear that community prevention pays off. But to see these results, we have to invest in the long game of community health. In America, pol-

> The community home visits significantly reduced criminal behavior in the women's offspring fifteen years later.

iticians talk about being "tough on crime." Instead, we need to be "gentle on new moms." Providing broader community and home support for moms will not only affect this generation, but generations down the line.

> In America, politicians talk about being "tough on crime." Instead, we need to be "gentle on new moms."

Advocates for mental health have adopted similar community care models. In 2018 one out of every five people (in the US and UK) were affected by some form of mental illness. In the US, that's 44.7 million people.[17] Kids are particularly impacted with rising rates of depression and suicide.[18] The absolute worst part is, half of adults and kids with mental illness don't seek treatment, and suicide takes eight hundred thousand lives a year globally.[19] The reason, in part, has to do with both stigma and fewer mental health resources.

Making things worse, mental health takes a back seat to physical health. In 2018, according to the WHO, only 1 percent of global aid went toward mental health.[20] Just a reminder that depression is the leading cause of ill health and disability worldwide.[21] It costs $1 trillion in lost productivity a year.[22] The WHO declares the prevalence of mental illness (13 percent) a far greater threat to global health than heart disease (10 percent), cancer (5 percent), or diabetes (1 percent).[23] While

> Depression is the leading cause of ill health and disability worldwide.

the investment in mental health treatment ultimately offsets the high societal cost, in the US in 2018, thirty-two states still didn't guarantee equal coverage for mental health care.[24] While all this data is discouraging, there is reason for hope, but it is going to take you and me getting involved.

In the US, the need for mental health services far outweighs the available resources. Working in mental health, I know how tough and expensive it can be to get an appointment with a psychiatrist or therapist. When crisis hits, it doesn't work to wait three weeks to see a medical professional. Plus, wouldn't it be better to prevent a crisis from happening in the first place? Dr. Gary Belkin, New York City's top mental health official told me that continuing to focus all our care and resources on the "black box" of a clinic or hospital "seems silly." After all, "99.99 percent of life and mental health happens outside the black box."[25]

This is where programs like Mental Health First Aid (#BeThe Difference) come in. Like Every Mother Counts, Mental Health First Aid trains people outside health care to make a difference. Peers, teachers, parents, neighbors, police officers, firefighters, office workers, and community leaders—you too can participate!—to safely provide initial support for a developing problem and/or to aid someone in crisis.

Learning Mental Health First Aid is like taking a CPR class—you may save a life. In the eight-hour course (usually taught in four-hour blocks over two days), participants learn to identify and respond to mental health challenges such as anxiety, depression, suicidal thoughts, substance use, and overdoses. To spread the word and train this new type of first responder, the National Council for Behavioral Health partnered with Born This Way Foundation—an organization started by singer Lady Gaga and her mom, Cynthia Germanotta, to empower young people to create a kinder and braver world.[26] Currently close to one million people across the US have been trained, including Michelle Obama, Dr. Oz, and Patrick Kennedy. Maybe you will join their ranks?

While you may never have heard of Alma-Ata, programs like Every Mother Counts and Mental Health First Aid (with Born This Way's help) are carrying forward its spirit: that it is our responsibility to take care of each other. Dr. Belkin and his team designed a program called Thrive NYC to train laypeople or peer health workers in preschools, churches, senior centers, community programs, and prisons to help address the city's unmet mental health needs. Other task-shifting programs are popping up for diabetes care and nutritional services.

Despite these gains, the vast potential behind the Alma-Ata Declaration, task-shifting programs, and the hidden factors remains untapped. What is it about the underlying message of caring for each other and helping out our neighbors that is so hard to adopt? What are we missing? And what are the tools that allow us to give and receive help? As we discussed, collective health is a dynamic two-way process between you (the individual) and the community. And at the heart of collective health is a solid bond of trust.

But trusting others is tough, especially when we feel we have good reason not to put our faith in them. We let our differences get in the way. We hunker down with like-minded individuals and build walls around our camps with an "us versus them" mind-set. And smoldering conflict erodes trust and goodwill.

When we feel distrustful and fearful that someone is out to get us, we're less inclined to work cooperatively with them, even when it's in our best interest. This behavior is well studied in economics. The "prisoner's dilemma" illustrates how acting in rational self-interest (doing something to the other guy before he does something to you) can backfire. The critical dilemma is that you have to trust your partners and cooperate to succeed. If we can trust one another and work together, we all stand to gain. When we distrust each other, we all stand to lose big time. Starting from our earliest civilizations, cooperation is the foundation of human society. Trust is also the foundation of health.

This means that unless we turn things around, we've got trouble.

Diminished trust in others means less willingness to invest in the common good and services that can benefit everyone. This includes schools, parks, roads, bridges, libraries, museums, fire departments, public safety, courts, clean air, clean water, health care, or the arts. Trust allows us to see that investing in other people is investing in ourselves. And this includes investing internationally as well. As a retired veteran who served in Afghanistan pointed out, imagine if armies with boots on the ground spent less time putting up barbed wire fences and more time building new schools. Maybe long-term occupations would result in a generation of scholars, not fighters. If we don't invest in common-good services for everyone, then we all miss out in the long term.

In the 1970s, about 60 percent of people (in the UK and America) agreed with the statement "Most other people can be trusted." By 2000 it was down to 30 percent.[27] In 2018 the Edelman Trust Barometer found that the US had the most precipitous drop in aggregate trust in eighteen years across institutions such as government, NGOs, and media.[28] This massive decline has big implications for our everyday lives because trust influences how people behave. When we're paranoid that the other guy is out to get us, it's hard to relax.

Feeling fearful and distrustful of those around us wears on us and physically alters our brains. It's like living with a lion. Once our primitive brain amygdala activates, our fear circuits override our ability to think clearly and problem-solve with our more collected cortex. Neuroscientists such as Dr. Wendy Suzuki from New York University have concluded that if we feel under threat on a daily basis, we start to lose brain volume in critical areas such as the temporal lobe and hippocampus, which diminishes our capacity to learn, create, and imagine.[29] (This is part of the reason that trust in school and work settings is so critical for problem-solving.)

Anger at unfairness may be hardwired. After all, monkeys are perfectly happy receiving cucumbers as payment for a small task, until one of them, in plain sight of the others, gets a grape. The gift of a grape to one lucky monkey sparks outrage among the others. They go bananas and are known to hurl cucumbers at the researcher in disdain over the injustice.[30] (A similar riot occurs if you bring mostly vanilla and only a few chocolate mini cupcakes to a preschool class. You've been warned.) It seems we can't help but compare ourselves and feel mad if we come up short.

The work of London School of Economics professor emeritus Lord Richard Layard indicates that diminished trust between us all, and the upset unfairness brings, contributes significantly to our poor mental health. The little girl described in the beginning of this chapter is all of us. When you or I feel good, we're more able to do good. We engage more proactively with each other. When conflict arises, we have the bandwidth to respond and not simply react. Feeling well facilitates problem-solving, trust, and collective reliance. On the flip side, when we're unhappy or fearful, we're less able to take care of others and contribute our part to the common good. Left unchecked, it becomes a vicious cycle. Which means we've got work to do.

To try to understand what we can do to rebuild our collective health, I spoke with Professor Layard.[31] Despite his intimidating title, at age eighty-four he retains the openness and youthful zest of a man on a mission. Well-known for his cheerful manner, innovative approaches to mental health, and kinship with the Dalai Lama, he's been given the

well-earned nickname of the UK's "happiness tsar." His research illuminates that the emphasis on the bottom line is missing the bigger picture
of what's important in life.

Research shows that despite significantly higher personal incomes
and skyrocketing national GDPs, human beings are not any happier
than they were fifty years ago.[32] All the evidence suggests that clinical depression has increased since the end of World War II.[33] As we discussed
in chapter 4, a threshold of money is helpful for health and well-being,
and that's why it is critical we help people out of abject poverty. But beyond a certain amount, there are no real gains in happiness. In the UK,
the variation in income only accounts for 1 percent of the variation in
happiness, and in no country is it more than 2 percent.[34] Much like the
health paradox, there is also a wealth paradox: as our incomes doubled,
our emotional well-being shrank.[35]

Professor Layard notes our singular misguided focus on money
promotes an "ultra-competitive environment where people excessively
worry about income, grades, and appearance." He suggests that instead
of focusing on working harder to make more money in hopes that happiness will follow, we need to turn our individual and collective attention
to achieving more happiness and emotional well-being.

Happiness isn't some sort of amorphous goal. It turns out, just asking
if a person feels good (or bad) can be measured along a reliable con-
tinuum across genders and countries. It also correlates with electrical
activity in different regions of the brain in studies done by Dr. Richard
Davidson at the University of Wisconsin-Madison, showing activation in
the left prefrontal cortex with positive feelings and activation in the right
prefrontal cortex with negative feelings.[36] And sustained enjoyment of
life only happens when we treat each other well.

When I asked Professor Layard how we get back on track to trust and
mutual respect, he replied, "We need a big culture change." As an individual, that sounds overwhelming, but he has a plan that might work. It
involves you, me, and the Dalai Lama.

To build global trust and collective health despite serious conflict,
we don't need to board a plane to Kazakhstan and sit in uncomfortable
seats in an imposing convention center. We can just sit at our kitchen

tables and start there. The first step is to focus on our own emotional well-being (ironic, isn't it?) so that we can contribute to a happier and kinder world.

Professor Layard is doing his part to address emotional well-being. In 2010 he teamed up with social innovator Geoff Mulgan, educator Sir Anthony Seldon, and the Dalai Lama to devise a plan called Action for Happiness. The global movement aims to refocus individuals—you and me—on committing to happier and more caring lives, not just richer ones. They gathered experts from a variety of fields including psychology, economics, education, neuroscience, technology, medicine, and public policy to use the evidence base to help boost individual and societal mental well-being. Mo Gawdat, founder of Moonshot for Humanity and #onebillionhappy, is helping out too. Millions of people around the world have signed up.

A quick way to boost happiness is to take positive action. As the maxim goes, "To feel good, do good." As a first step, you can take a pledge on Action for Happiness's website (http://www.actionforhappiness.org) to commit to being a force for good, which I did. It reads simply, "I will try to create more happiness and less unhappiness in the world around me."[37] The idea is we can each contribute to a happier world in our homes, schools, workplaces, and neighborhoods. In other words, opportunities await us in all the hidden areas that we have discussed in this book. We can task ourselves to live with more compassion and expand social trust.

Action for Happiness has already made impressive headway. As well as building a huge global community of supporters, their founders have helped establish model mental health programs in Britain to begin to tackle treatment gaps, suicide, and loneliness. The UK even launched a loneliness strategy in 2017 and appointed its first Minister of Loneliness to directly address this massive mental health need. Even the OECD, or club of rich nations, has recently adopted happiness measures such as GNH (Gross National Happiness) to move beyond money as the global measure of success.

On a local level, Action for Happiness created an eight-week course, called "Exploring What Matters." The class meets in small groups once a week. It's a time for individuals to tune in, connect face-to-face, and take action. It uses scientific evidence to frame topics such as adversity, relationships, and improving our workplaces and communities. During meetings, people share their experiences, and at the end, participants chose how they will act on what they learned that week, like reaching out to a neighbor or chatting with someone in front of them in line at the store.[38] Small gestures with profound consequences. People who complete the course get a bigger happiness boost than those who get a job after being unemployed. They also become more compassionate and more trusting of others. After speaking to Professor Layard, I volunteered to facilitate a group in New York. Maybe you will start one in your hometown too.

One terrific idea that came from an "Exploring What Matters" group is the Happy Café Network, with locations popping up around the world in the UK, Canada, Costa Rica, Taiwan, Australia, and more. The café is simply a designation via a sticker in the window for a welcoming place where patrons can talk with others interested in improving well-being.[39] It can take place in coffee shops, community centers, houses of worship, libraries, or schools—basically any common gathering place where activities help people share their stories, feel inspired, and connect with others. The idea is to leave feeling better than when you arrived. Layard believes that happiness comes down to our social connections, which these cafés promote. "In the end, it's face-to-face relationships that give the ultimate satisfaction," he says. Engaging in conversations where we feel heard and respected helps us relax, build trust, create positive connection and psychological safety.

Group activities can help create a safe space and expand your circle of trust whether you join an "Exploring What Matters" course, a Happy Café, meet-ups for parents, group therapy, a writing club, chorus, Quaker-style listening circle, a women's business collective, basketball league, running club, or fitness class. (One of my favorites is SoulCycle, which aims to create a safe emotional space for riders, and I've heard instructors fearlessly share their own traumas and experiences overcoming adversity.) When you start to look, multiple forms of engaging participation exist where you can feel a connection to others, build psychological safety, and discuss shared experiences. Starting at orientation in medical school, I was assigned a "small group" of about ten classmates to talk to about our hopes and fears. While we all regularly met for the first month with a faculty preceptor and senior student as part of the formal curriculum, we informally continued to meet for years, oftentimes at lunch and occasionally at evening potlucks. It was an invaluable part of training and a huge reason I loved medical school.

Groups boost solidarity in part because of something known as consciousness-raising. This grassroots idea has a history in the civil rights movement, labor organizing, and the women's movement.[40] Togetherness raises awareness that you are not alone. It validates your experience and that you do not deserve to feel mocked or "crazy." An earnest conversation can generate change in group participants through the "four A's"—awareness, acceptance, absorption, and action. This is usually facilitated in part by a group leader, which is particularly helpful when a fifth "A"—anger—shows up.

Groups that move beyond griping alone help us metabolize anger and rebuild trust in other people in the face of trauma. Professor Layard says he's found over his long lifetime that "anger does not lead to a good outcome, but solidarity is important." So if we create a sanctuary to acknowledge feelings and experiences, even the big hairy ugly ones, it can help boost emotional well-being, foster solidarity with others, and craft collective health.

Achieving solidarity requires us to strengthen our conflict-resolution skills. A basic part of trust is the ability to acknowledge our differences and deal peacefully with disagreements when they arise. Conflict is an inevitable part of daily life in our countries and our homes. According to one survey of two thousand parents of children age two to twelve, the average household argues for over eight minutes, six times a day.[41] In my family, with three young boys who all want to play with the same exact toy at the same exact time, it feels like closer to every two seconds. But I remind myself that learning to resolve conflict is an incredibly valuable skill that takes daily practice. Our whole lives, we are always learning to do it better.

Dr. King and other peacemakers, such as Gandhi, believed every human being could use the tools of conflict resolution to create a more loving society. Dr. King saw violence as a learned behavior. He also saw that we can train ourselves to find other solutions to our differences. He said, "The choice is not between violence and nonviolence but between violence and non-existence." Peace studies teach that violence doesn't usually come out of nowhere. It stems from unaddressed and unresolved conflicts that boil over and then create a huge mess.

After college in the late 1990s, I lived in Washington, DC. I had so little money that my big Sunday luxury was eating out at the corner fast-food burrito place, where I would overindulge in the condiment and salsa bar. One night, some friends and I came across a free evening seminar called "Solutions to Violence" taught by journalist and peace studies teacher extraordinaire Colman McCarthy. At the time, DC had a reputation as the nation's "murder capital." We all worked and/or lived in neighborhoods that had experienced a lot of violence, and we'd all repeatedly heard the *pop, pop, pop* of gunfire ringing out in the capital city. The class offered a glimmer of understanding of how we might help.

McCarthy himself is an inspiration. After a long career at the *Washington Post*, including assignments to interview multiple Nobel Peace Prize winners such as Mother Teresa and Nelson Mandela, he decided in 1982 to dedicate his time to teaching courses on peace and conflict resolution in public high schools, local universities, and community centers. Even at eighty, he is still often seen biking among all his different teaching posts. More than twenty years after I took his seminar, I still look at my tattered notebook and wonder how we all can cast such an ever-widening circle for peace and joy.

Imagine if every one of us learned to navigate conflict skillfully. How different would our homes, schools, workplaces, neighborhoods, communities, and nations look? It is going to take all of us to keep our planet healthy in the decades ahead. Earth has some big environmental challenges on the horizon, so we're going to need to put aside our differences and problem-solve together. And it starts at home. Like the little girl I described in the beginning of this chapter, what a relief it would be if we could feel that others had our back and would help us negotiate conflict. This form of psychological trust forms the foundation of the Beloved Community. As McCarthy said, "Being a pacifist doesn't mean being passive. It means being a peacemaker."[42] In his seminar, which he has now taught for thirty-seven years to well over ten thousand students, he explains key conflict-resolution skills, partly inspired by Gandhi and Dr. King. I have listed some of them here, with my own experiences in the mix:

1. **Name the conflict.** Amazingly, three out of four people who are fighting are mad about different issues. So make sure you understand the actual matter at hand and gather needed information to increase understanding of the problem. When walking into a conflict in the ER, I learned from top hospital security to always start by asking, "What's the problem here?" rather than "What happened?" which can trigger the blame game and flare tempers.

2. **It's not you versus me. It's you and me versus the problem.** For instance, in America, it's not red versus blue states. It's all of us seeking common ground. Conflict resolution is about defeating unjust systems, forces, policies, and acts—but not people.[43] In other words, you aren't trying to humiliate the opposition, but solve the problem together. Civil rights leaders such as Dr. King and Congressman John Lewis also taught that if the other side chooses to ignore the problem or remove themselves from the discussion, you need to creatively find a way to keep on the moral pressure for engagement. (Such as riding buses and sitting at lunch counters.)

3. **Find a neutral place to hold the conversation.** In a school, it could be a "peace room" with designated peer mediators, or in a home, a "peace table" where conflicts are solved. In a Manhattan-size apartment, we often form a listening circle on the floor, Native American style. The key is to shift from the battleground mind-set to using the more rational cortex.

4. **Listen more than you speak.** When tensions are escalating, participants need to feel that they have an opportunity to be fairly heard. To facilitate, a "talking stick" from Native Amer-

ican traditions helps. (In our family meetings, we often use a stuffed animal or the remote control in place of an actual stick.) Only the person who is holding the stick can talk, and he can continue until he feels he has made his point. Others are only allowed to ask clarifying questions. Tensions often dramatically decrease once someone knows that he has the space to be heard. (Best to establish the ground rules of these meetings before tempers flare.)

5. **List out shared concerns and needs.** Addressing the problem together helps build cooperation. Using skills such as grace and humor during this process leaves the door open to see the good in the other side.

6. **Start with one small, doable action.** To problem-solve big issues, take one manageable step to address the problem and then build momentum from there. Trying to address too much too soon is a recipe for a fiasco. As an expert social worker in the ER taught me, politely remind an angry person who might be making unreasonable demands that you can't give him what you don't have.

7. **Practice forgiveness.** Forgiveness is different than being right or wrong. You can disagree with someone's actions and still forgive. (This makes me think of Congressman Lewis accepting an apology from a man who beat him bloody decades earlier during a civil rights march. Lewis not only forgave him, but the man and his son visited Lewis multiple times afterward.)[44] Label actions and behaviors, not people, as good or bad. The idea is that letting go of vengeance allows peace of mind and an opportunity to move forward. The ultimate goals of conflict resolution are friendship, understanding, and reconciliation. Otherwise, the cycle of conflict just continues underground. Also, you must create opportunities for people to redeem themselves.

8. **Treat yourself with compassion.** McCarthy, Dr. King, and Gandhi echo the message of Professor Layard, the Dalai Lama, and this book: if you tend to your emotional well-being and happiness (and get a good night's sleep to boot), you'll be far better equipped to deal with conflicts and stand up to advocate for others.[45]

Life gives us multiple teaching moments to practice these skills with the goal of making these habits instinctual. And by doing so, you'll begin to actively see instances of injustice that go on around you. Because sometimes if they're not happening to you, you're not attuned to them. And even when you are, you may feel it's not your place to get involved. But standing up and calling out injustice is essential in the Beloved Community. I'm reminded of a third grader on the playground who heard his friend being called "stupid" by some fifth-grade boys they were playing ball with. He told the kids, "Hey, that's not nice." When the kids didn't respond and continued taunting, he found the children's grown-ups and told them. The grown-ups thankfully listened and addressed the issue. That child's bravery allowed the game to resume, minus the name-calling.

Imagine if we all had the courage to speak up against unkindness in playgrounds, schools, and workplaces. If left unaddressed, bullying, lies, and wrongdoing start to seem acceptable and sever the threads of the fabric of society. But if just one brave person turns a flashlight on injustice, we are no longer in the dark. And we are no longer alone. By speaking out, we validate each other's experience and create a ripple effect of courage and trust. We can repair and strengthen our collective health by speaking up for one another.

I discovered the power of one voice at an unlikely place: a beauty store makeup counter. In February 2018, preparing for a presentation, I decided to take a break and buy myself some lipstick, something I rarely do. In the tiny Benefits cosmetics store, a staff member asked if I would mind sitting for a cosmetology student. The trainee was a petite young woman with dark shoulder-length hair; soulful, wise eyes; and a disarmingly calm manner. The staff member introduced her as Nadia. While I had things to do, I agreed. When I sat on the barstool, I still towered over her slight frame. The seemingly shy young woman spoke very little as I closed my eyes and she gently ran brushes over my face, getting directions from her seasoned instructor. "Yes! Yes! She needs more coverage there, and there, and waaaaaaay more there! More!!!!"

With my eyes still closed, I asked Nadia about studying to become a makeup artist. I learned her dream was to one day open a beauty shop to help women feel strong and beautiful. Yes, makeup can feel empowering, and as we know from chapter 2, the caring touch a beautician can provide is bonding and critical for human beings' health. We also know, from chapter 3, that beauty shops provide an important setting for social connection as well.

As we talked, I got the impression that Nadia didn't live in New York. I learned she grew up in a small town in Iraq. The makeup instructor explained that she was visiting for the day and *Glamour* magazine had sponsored her training. Okay. He then added, "Nadia escaped slavery." *What?* I opened my eyes as he continued, "Amal Clooney was her lawyer." I next learned how the quiet young woman before me had bravely raised her voice in the dark. When others felt shamed into silence or could not speak for themselves, she spoke for them.

On the night of August 3, 2014, when Nadia Murad was twenty-one years old, Islamic militants ambushed her quiet farming community of Kocho. Six of her brothers were executed that night. She and her two sisters, along with the other young women and girls in her village, were held hostage, separated, and sold into slavery. She never saw her funny and smart sixty-one-year-old mother again, who was reportedly killed for being too old to sell. Over the three months of captivity that followed, Nadia was repeatedly raped and tortured.[46] When she tried to escape and failed, she was severely beaten and raped by a group of her captors in an attempt to humiliate her. When she did narrowly escape and made it to safety, rather than stay quiet, she chose to share her story. She felt it was her duty to help the thousands of women and children who remain enslaved and subjected to ongoing sexual violence. She also knew she discussed something "so painful and private" at great personal risk.[47] But she did it anyway. She pledged to be a voice not just for the Yazidi people of her homeland, but for the countless victims of war and sexual violence around the world.

Nadia wrote a book about her experience called *The Last Girl: My Story of Captivity, My Fight Against the Islamic State.*[48] Amal Clooney invited her to speak at the United Nations on behalf of survivors. Finally, in September 2017, the UN passed a resolution to investigate the crimes against the Yazidi people in Iraq.[49] Nadia hopes to raise awareness of ongoing violence toward women around the world, hold those accountable who commit offenses, achieve justice for survivors, and rebuild communities ravaged by genocide. "We must support efforts to focus on humanity, and overcome political and cultural divisions," she said. In short, we must start "prioritizing humanity, not war."[50] Nadia's brave words and actions echoed Dr. King's Beloved Community. When the makeup instructor took a photo of us, I realized I was the student of Nadia's unwavering courage.

As life rolled on, over a half a year later, I heard that the committee for the Nobel Peace Prize had announced the 2018 winners, so I googled to see who had won. I stared at the photo that popped up and the unwavering soulful, wise eyes that looked back at me. Sure enough, Nadia had received the award, the second youngest recipient ever, along with Dr. Denis Mukwege from the Democratic Republic of the Congo, who survived an assassination attempt for helping rape survivors, denouncing the ongoing conflict in his country, and calling for justice at the UN.[51] Both showed fearless bravery in using their voices to end the use of sexual violence as a weapon of war and get women the help they deserve.

While bombs don't kill ideas, words can. Nadia says she tells her story because it is her best weapon against shame.[52] Her courage has inspired countless others to stand up for human rights, justice, and peace. I hope it will inspire you to stand up too. As Colman McCarthy said, "Studying peace through nonviolence is as much about getting the bombs out of our world as it is about getting them out of our heart."[53] Nadia's courage to address ongoing conflict takes us all a step closer to collective health.

As we've seen throughout this book, our health primarily depends on our social world and investment in the common good. Our bonds of trust hold it together. A key part of building trust is that we attend to our own emotional well-being so that when conflict arises, we can find the courage to respond effectively and communicate fearlessly. Imagine if each of us committed to looking out for one another, speaking out against injustice, and navigating our differences peacefully. Our voices in harmony reach those who feel alone and remind us all that there is a fundamental goodness we can all tap into. In this virtuous circle, our individual actions boost collective health for everyone. The Beloved Community begins with each of us. Your voice matters just like Nadia's. As we'll see in the conclusion, your daily actions can create a ripple effect for peace.

The Ripple Effect:
Getting to Kindness

Each time a man stands up for an ideal, or acts to improve the lot of others, or strikes out against injustice, he sends forth a tiny ripple of hope, and crossing each other from a million different centers of energy and daring, those ripples build a current which can sweep down the mightiest walls of oppression and resistance.
—ROBERT F. KENNEDY

Kindness gives birth to kindness.
—SOPHOCLES

What will it take to make us well?

Let's go back to the beginning of our journey and how we define health and well-being. In this book's early pages, I said that I wanted to empower you to change your health, but not in the usual ways. I promised I wouldn't give you a ten-step fitness plan or a two-week diet. Wellness extends far beyond these quick fixes or piecemeal measures. Plus, it is way more fun than eating a bunch of kale alone.

As we've roamed the halls of the hospital together exploring clinical puzzles and journeyed through the hidden factors of health, I hope you've come to see that spending more on medical care alone will not make us healthier. The puzzle pieces laid out side by side reveal a stunning picture. Total health extends far beyond biomedicine. If we want to better our health, we need a larger, more panoramic view of health.

By now, that larger, more inclusive picture is coming into focus. Starting with Murina Levesque, the caring postdoc who tended the white rabbits, health isn't about just what's happening in the body or our cholesterol levels. True wellness is more than our physical health, and it begins far before we land in the hospital; it includes our relationships, jobs, education, purpose, housing, and neighborhoods. It is also about fairness and policies that promote a healthy and safe environment for everyone.

Health is right there with us when we hold a baby, call our sister, or hang out with friends bowling. Health joins us when we sit in a meeting at work, or crack open a book on our couch, or plant tulips in a flower box. It also meets us when we speak out against injustice and look out for a child's welfare. Or when we lend a hand to the person in front of us. Health is found in glimmers of kindness and the comforts of love, respect, and safety. True health is hidden in the million tiny moments of our everyday lives.

This book has focused on how our social world becomes a part of us and powerfully shapes our mental and physical health. But we also shape our social world. It's now clear that the model of the hidden factors of health introduced in chapter 1 is not static. Instead, it's an interactive fluid system: one in which we all participate during every waking moment of our lives. Our impact even continues to reverberate long after we are gone.

The hug we give our spouse or child as we walk out the door in the morning may influence how he handles an unpleasant interaction at work or school. The friendly chat with a neighbor may help her be kinder to the man behind the register where she buys her coffee on her commute to work. If we offer encouraging or demeaning feedback to an employee, it may sway whether she decides to attend a night class to feed her brain or chooses to veg out in front of the TV after work. It may also influence how she treats her family when she arrives home, which may in turn affect their stress levels that evening. Ultimately, these simple actions add up to how well we all sleep at night. Which affects our health. And starts the cycle anew the next morning.

Think of it this way.

Each small daily choice we make nurtures our emotional well-being or aggravates our stress in a way that helps or hinders our physical health. Repeated decisions that support our emotional well-being buffer the negative stress that inevitably shows up during the course of a day and a lifetime. We can build up our reserves of health or deplete them. It's a bit like the butterfly effect (or the 1998 movie *Sliding Doors*). Even the smallest change in our behavior can ripple outward with consequences for much larger events down the road. This is the spillover of the social multiplier effect. It shows how there is great power in starting with a friendly "hello."

On a daily basis, our small, seemingly insignificant choices and experiences create the cultural fabric of something so much grander than we ever imagined. No human being exists in a vacuum. In a continual ebb and flow, every one of our actions in the hidden factors creates a vast unseen ripple effect (see figure 6) with profound consequences for not just our health, but everyone's.

Here is what I wish I had known when I was starting in medical school and life: our social conditions (hidden factors) profoundly shape our physical and mental health. Kind and loving choices that support emotional well-being and reduce stress may help prevent or delay the onset of many diseases. As we've discussed, ample evidence shows that toxic or prolonged stress increases inflammation, shortens telomeres, and alters epigenetics, which puts a person at risk of heart attack, stroke, infection, cancer, diabetes, mental illnesses, osteoporosis, autoimmune disorders, and premature death. The contrary is also true. The more buffers for negative stress we create, the healthier we are, even with diseases that may come. While death is inevitable, the essentials of health allow us to live as healthy as possible on our journey.

And it's not only our own health or susceptibility to disease that's in question in this broader definition of health. Because if I'm creating buffers for my stress—and I'm doing that by playing basketball with you or voting for our neighborhood to have more green parks and better lights

THE RIPPLE EFFECT:
A DYNAMIC MODEL OF HIDDEN FACTORS

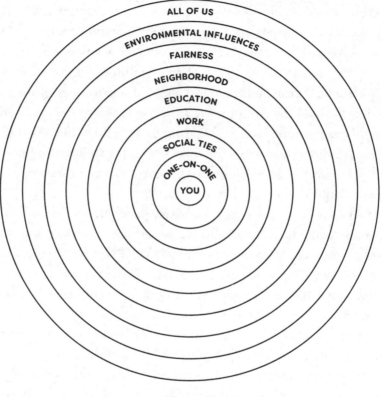

ALL OF US

ENVIRONMENTAL INFLUENCES

FAIRNESS

NEIGHBORHOOD

EDUCATION

WORK

SOCIAL TIES

ONE-ON-ONE

YOU

Figure 5

or treating you the way I would want to be treated—I'm simultaneously addressing your negative stress and building our collective health. In this dynamic model, how I act in the world affects others and how others act affects you. Our emotional health is thus collectively and not just individually shaped. Which brings us to kindness. While our clever brains may trick us into thinking we are in this for ourselves, the evidence shows we are all in this together.

To see the ripple effect of health in action, let's go back to Bella from chapter 1. Three years out from a pancreatic cancer diagnosis, she was living a full life. While something had gone awry at the cellular, tissue, and organ level, on a personal level she thrived. To be clear, her life was not perfect. Nobody's ever is. But she had significant buffers through her social interactions that protected her in times of stress. As we have seen, true health is most often tested in how someone lives with a disease.

At the time of Bella's cancer diagnosis, things had gotten rough. Life had delivered a one-two punch. Her longtime partner, Greta, had died earlier that year in a freak rock climbing accident several hours north from their Westchester, New York, home. The pair had met decades before in law school. Greta had always been extremely athletic and was an experienced climber. On that sunny September morning, somehow her harness malfunctioned and the belay loop snapped. While the grief felt unbearable, Bella had the support of her adult son, Toby, his father (Bella's best friend), her sister and niece, a host of cousins, a tight group of friends from law school, and colleagues from her career in public law to get her through the initial shock. Her years of nurturing these relationships carried her through her darkest nights, much as she had supported them over the years.

Thankfully, well before Greta died, Bella had become active at the local community center in their neighborhood. She felt lucky to have the center nearby and to have well-tended, well-lit sidewalks to get there and back, even in winter. Bella met many friends through her painting and writing classes. After Greta died, Bella used her writing as a way to still feel connected to her. When Bella was diagnosed with pancreatic cancer, she used her painting to distract herself during her cancer treatment. Her positive attitude, kindness, and courage inspired the others she met at the center as they faced their own challenges.

In the hospital, where I met Bella, she became a beloved patient. She often brought friends, family, or neighbors with her to chemo and once showed up with candy necklaces for the staff. The staff, in turn, always seemed more chipper and kinder to the other patients when she was around. Although she must have felt physically drained, she somehow managed to make something unpleasant seem like a party. She became active in a cancer support group and, with her son Toby's help, encouraged the local organization to bolster their family support programs. She noted that while she never would have wished for Greta's death or getting the cancer diagnosis, she felt an intensified appreciation of life and spirituality after these experiences. She also inspired me by defying her original prognosis of only six months to live.

The last update I heard was that Bella had outlived her oncologist.

Bella's story illustrating the ripple effect shows how interactions in her hidden factors promoted health even with adversity. It's easy to appreciate how the ripples are dynamic and can become hard to tease apart in practice because they overlap in multiple ways. As an individual, Bella exceeded in giving and received kindness, love, and support. She also brought with her a sense of creativity, spunk, and warmth. Bella abundantly returned back to the world the support she'd received, creating even more ripples of well-being and harmony for others.

One night while I was reading a bedtime story to my three boys, Ryan, who was then six, looked at me intently. The line I'd finished was, "Heart-prints can heal us with the power of love."[1] Ryan pushed his red hair out of his eyes and leaned in for a closer look at the page. The cartoon drawings showed a girl sick in bed, covered with mysterious red bumps, who stands up smiling after her friend visits. Ryan also sat in his bed covered head to toe with spots his pediatrician assured us were caused by a virus. "Mommy, love isn't going to take away my rash. It just isn't." It was my turn to pause.

It's true that love doesn't magically—poof—clear up a rash, heal a broken bone, or cure cancer. But research shows it is the hidden context of health, and every human body tells its story. Studying the hidden factors and their ripple effect, we know kindness and connection help prevent disease and reduce illness severity. And here's the amazing thing: to cultivate relationships, contribute to our communities, and be kind costs nothing. We each have the capability to contribute to better health for others and ourselves. But we do need the will. Looking for others who promote kindness, fairness, and compassion can inspire action.

On West Twelfth Street, a tree-lined block of Greenwich Village in

New York City, there is a large multicolored sign that sits in front of a well-tended brownstone. The hand-painted words read, "If we all do one random act of kindness a day, we might just set the world in the right direction." I see this sign daily at home. Once, in a waiting room, I found copies of it mixed in with magazines. I hung it on the back of my family's door as a daily parting reminder.

When I started working on this book, I asked to meet with the sign's artist, Marty Kornfeld. My eldest son, Max, then eight, joined me. Marty, who looks the part of an artist with a mop of blond hair, a trim gray beard, minimalist clothes, and an unaffected manner, told us that his mom inspired the message. She required Marty and his siblings to do at least two random acts of kindness daily. The gestures didn't need fanfare. Small kindnesses counted, such as lending a hand to a person carrying groceries, saying good morning to a neighbor, or offering a compliment. The task simply had to involve consideration passing from one person to another. If he returned home without having completed his mission, his mom sent him out again. Marty gave me a stack of posters like the one we had hanging at home and asked us to distribute them. We did. I offered copies to coworkers, and my kids gave then to classmates. Distributing them became a game. The copy I discovered in a waiting room years before probably had similar origins. Marty Kornfeld, in his unique way, makes positive waves.

As we left that day, Marty gave Max some paint samples to use to make his own art. At home, Max took a big sheet of paper and painted a big bright sun and lovely beach scene. Initially disappointed that blue paint was not among the colors provided, Max used his creativity to find a solution. He worked around the constraints to make the picture he dreamed. Max told me, "You can't see the ocean directly. It is just there on the other side of the sand dunes." Marty's gift, combined with Max's ingenuity, reminded me of the ripple effect, and how one good deed can spark others' imaginations.

Great movements often start where you least expect: with one person's courageous actions at the local level. Rosa Parks's decision to remain seated at the front of the bus in Montgomery, Alabama, created a ripple of change still being realized decades later across America. Standing up to injustice and questioning the status quo one person at a time takes tremendous courage, and it signals to others that they are not alone. As we discussed in chapter 10, positive personal choices inspire others to act and foster bonds of interconnectedness. From these bonds, a network is formed that becomes bigger than the individual—like a mass of sparrows flying in formation over a pasture. Every person unknowingly plays a part in health through her daily choices and opportunities to show kindness and speak out against injustice. Dr. Deepak Chopra said, "Humanity is one family. There is no us versus them." Our health and well-being depend on individuals making an effort in the tiny moments of daily life to strengthen the bonds between us.

Every morning, Benjamin Franklin would reportedly ask, "What good can I do today?" Or as my son Max, at age ten, asked after hearing about yet another school shooting, "Mom, why can't the world just be a little kinder? Why?" While policies that protect people and keep schools safe help, it starts with individual actions. What if everyone practiced everyday friendliness, or microkindnesses? In day-to-day interactions—a person looking lost, a screaming child, an angry customer—a person can ask, *What can I do at this moment that could add kindness to the situation?* It may mean stopping to give someone directions, offering a hug or a smile, or listening. Small gestures that support human worth practiced regularly create community and foster trust. Acting with respect, compassion, patience, humor, and generosity is good for the doer and the receiver. And in doing that, we not only build our own health but our collective health. In microkindnesses, there is great strength.

Let's be clear that being kind takes bravery. It requires standing fearless and doesn't mean being passive or being a pushover. There are people, most notably some men in positions of power, who view kindness as a weakness to manipulate. They may try to shut down meaningful conversation in the name of civility, but they are mistaken. Genuine kindness takes a strong will to hear someone else out. Shutting

Being kind takes bravery. It requires standing fearless and doesn't mean being passive or being a pushover.

down conversation because you don't like what the other side has to say is not civil discourse. You and I may not agree, but we can still listen to each other and have a respectful discussion. In fact, it is critical that we make the space to hear one another out in our communities, homes, and our nation.

Kindness also means acknowledging our own and others' anger and channeling it into positive action and coalitions. It means recognizing someone else's pain and trauma and trying to understand where they are coming from. By listening, we can respect others' experience and design solutions together to do something about the situation. And what's amazing is that when leaders fail to hear us, we can listen to each other as individuals. Our individual actions leave ripples on the people around us. As more people create positive ripples, the bigger the amplitude. Together we can create a groundswell of powerful positive change.

Once one understands that society is more than half the story of health, it becomes apparent that one doesn't need a white coat, a fancy degree, or anyone's permission to improve health today. While individuals can take a daily stand to practice microkindnesses and ask, "What good can I do today?" so, too, can organizations and companies. There are numerous opportunities within everyone's scope of influence to build community and expand circles of trust. Inspirational stories of groups making a difference—Meals on Wheels, (RED), Girls Who Code, Born This Way Foundation, the Ice Bucket Challenge, Beyond Differences, God's Love We Deliver, charity: water, Gilda's Club, CLIMB, debra, Every Mother Counts, Smart Girls, and countless others—show how support and connection foster health during adversity. Beyond nonprofit programs, companies can also make positive social ripples. Examples are numerous and include corporations such as Google, the Walt Disney Company, Starbucks, Ben & Jerry's, TOMS, Patagonia, Microsoft, IKEA, Nike, Warby Parker, SoulCycle, and Lego. While the names of the companies will undoubtedly change with time, the spirit of inclusivity and tolerance that inspire action will remain. Ordinary individuals, groups, and businesses, not only doctors or hospitals, can improve global health. We can do so much better together.

While living back home in Nevada after college, I applied for and got a yearlong AmeriCorps experience as a peer health educator in Washington, DC. It was transformative. Each week from Monday to Thursday, I worked in a free clinic and delivered meals to homebound people with HIV/AIDS all over the city. I saw firsthand how people with serious illness lived in their homes. On Fridays, my AmeriCorps team and I would do community service projects in the DC area, from teaching school kids about health issues to clothing drives and park cleanups to rebuilding homes and helping out communities after disasters. If we could imagine it, we'd partner with other people in the area to make it a reality.

Kevin Kelly, cofounder of *Wired* magazine, said in an interview with Tim Ferriss that he'd make travel or time outside one's local community a requirement for all young people.[2] While I did not grow up with much money, my AmeriCorps experience was eye-opening to the extreme poverty and disparities surrounding our nation's capital. Working on a team of volunteers with different backgrounds from all over the country, I started to wrestle with my own assumptions. The experience undoubtedly helped me be a better doctor and planted the seeds that grew into this book. My AmeriCorps program alone, through the Washington AIDS Partnership (led by the amazing J. Channing Wickham), over twenty years provided 1.2 billion hours of public service. Investment in programs like AmeriCorps, Teach For America, the Peace Corps, Global Health Corps, and Senior Corps builds community, tolerance, and understanding. They, like other cultural exchange programs such as Fulbright Fellowships, are the training ground for a kinder, more civil society, which we now know is the foundation of health.

From schools like Sandy Hook Elementary and Stoneman Douglas High School to Paris, Orlando, Dallas, Las Vegas, San Bernardino, Pittsburgh, to refugee camps and a divided America, the world needs your kindness and understanding. In the time that I've written this book, the list of places and people who have known heartache has expanded exponentially. Unfortunately, as is probably clear to you, the ripple effect on our stress levels works negatively as well. Anger goes viral too.

But there is reason for hope.

I see hope when a mother holds her child. I see hope when one boy helps another who has fallen at the playground. I see hope when a young woman volunteers in an after-school enrichment program. I see hope when a group of teenagers gets engaged in national politics. I see hope when women will not tolerate harassment or discrimination in their workplace. I see hope when you finish this book and decide to take positive action too. The vast majority of us want healthy lives for our loved ones and ourselves. As the majority, we can't sit back in our bubbles hoping someone else will champion the cause. Health is not going to happen at our doctor's office alone. We must do this together in our communities, starting now.

Dr. Martin Luther King Jr. wrote, "Darkness cannot drive out darkness; only light can do that. Hate cannot drive out hate; only love can do that." Together we can all take steps to buffer ourselves better and nurture our well-being. We can also drive out the vortex of fear. I invite you to join the global community fostering fairness, kindness, and human dignity and share stories about your ripple effect on social media.

Our daily decisions can bring about powerful change in our lives, and the lives of those around us. To live a truly healthy life, we need to choose to connect to one other and find purpose, joy, and meaning in our lives. Each daily decision is an opportunity to honor human worth and kinship, and to act with love. A global movement can start locally with you, in your community, having important conversations about the hidden factors of health and our shared humanity. Collectively, we have the means to make it better for everyone. Kindness and love, after all, are abundant renewable resources. I think about this a lot. Throughout my three children's lifetimes, much will change. But one thing will remain constant in the ripple effect of health: the centrality of love.

The Enduring Mystery

*The total number of minds in the universe is one . . . Quantum
physics thus reveals a basic oneness of the universe.*
—ERWIN SCHRÖDINGER,
NOBEL PRIZE–WINNING PHYSICIST

As a doctor, I'm amazed by the magic math of the body: the sum is always far more than the parts alone. It reminds me of how during World War I, movie film footage was melted down for the chemical components. Fundamentally, film is simply silver and celluloid, but thinking of it that way misses the magic of cinema. Similarly, it's mind-boggling how a person's life far exceeds his body. Medicine's narrow focus on the parts ignores the bigger picture, the wonder of a human life.

Dr. John T. Hansen, my anatomy instructor, handed out lined white index cards the first week of medical school. He stood at the front of the lecture hall in his long white lab coat and called out each student by name. Since he was also the director of admissions, Dr. Hansen knew everyone's backstory. I was a political science major in college and a latecomer to medicine, and I felt he'd taken a chance on me. One by one, we scuttled down in our short white coats to the front of the room. "Kelli Jane Harding." With an earnest gaze through his rimless glasses (just like the ones my dad wore), he handed me a long-awaited invitation to a new world. I'd worked hard to arrive at that moment, and I didn't want to let him or myself down. The card read: "Table 9: Paul, Factory Worker. Cause of Death: Carcinoma of the Lung." My first patient.

That day, with uncomfortable laughter, my three lab partners—Omesh, Ed, and Abby—and I departed from a world of familiar social boundaries. After all, it's not every day you hang out with a dead body. Ed and Omesh were charming, funny, and smart. Abby entered medical school after a successful tech career on the West Coast. She brought a quiet worldly wit to our foursome. Fear makes fast friends, and thankfully we all shared a similar sense of humor. We barely knew one another's names to start, but by the end of our course many months later, we'd shared the strange and intimate experience of holding a human heart and brain in our hands.

Medical school anatomy isn't just the memorization of all the body's bits. It's the initiation into medicine. Once you see it, you can never unsee it. You laugh at things that you can't tell the uninitiated because you'd sound like a horrible person. The anatomy professor is crucial in shaping students' values in medicine: teamwork, responsibility, humility, and dignity above all else.[1] Dr. Hansen's flawless mix of unwavering professionalism and kindness upheld the best ideals of the field. After all, there's a fine line between anatomy lab and the actions of the criminally insane.

An engraved sign on the anatomy lab door read Authorized Personnel Only. That first day, I felt a chill when I realized that Authorized Personnel referred to me. The anatomy lab door mirrors the barrier between the worlds of the doctor and the patient: the divide is flimsy at best. Once inside, staff warned us to come into the room quickly and "never, ever prop the door open." Just up the hall was the anatomical gift office, where community members donate their bodies to science—perhaps the most exceptional kindness of all. I imagined a well-heeled woman walking by the lab on her way to the room, unaware that behind the door I stood sawing a pelvis in half with a chainsaw. Best to keep it closed.

The chilly room held twenty waist-high silver lab tables in evenly spaced rows. The donors lay on top of the tables covered in white sheets. I found table 9 with my team. The cloud of formaldehyde made me queasy. As medical students learn, the embalming fluid also curiously induces hunger. Over the months that followed, I grew less aware of the smell and far more conscious of my stomach rumbling. Many years later, I still can't open a package for a new plastic shower curtain laced with formaldehyde without thinking about Paul and a burrito.

The ritual the first day is to meet the donor before any dissection begins. My group chose to remove the small white cloth on his face. The face remains covered during the dissection; but this was a moment to acknowledge the person's humanity. The introduction serves as a reminder to align our actions going forward with the intention of the human being who gave us his most precious gift. In the months ahead, we'd concentrate so intently on slicing through tissues searching out nerves, arteries, and veins that we'd temporarily forget Paul, the person. Humanity took a back seat with an exam on the horizon.

That morning, the four of us stood silently beside a man we'd never get to thank. In a flash, we saw Paul's thick white hair, Roman nose, and handsome features. He looked younger than I'd expected, only in his sixties. Other than my grandpa Jack, my mom's dad, Paul's was the first dead body I'd seen. The tissues that composed Paul were intact, but it was immediately apparent that Paul the person was long gone. Like a smooth shell found on the beach, the body remained a token acknowledgment of the life that once resided there. I felt acutely aware of life in its absence. Vanished. The human essence or being or spark was absent. I couldn't help but wonder, *Where did the spark go? Where had it come from?* We quickly covered his face again. It would remain so throughout the rest of the semester until several months later, when the time came to dissect the head and brain. By that point, our indoctrination to medicine had sufficiently broken down our sense of common decency.

Like a smooth shell found on the beach, the body remained a token acknowledgment of the life that once resided there.

Despite all the detailed dissection that followed, including the neural networks that formed Paul's squishy three-pound brain, we never found Paul the person. Traces of freckles indicated he liked the outdoors. Laugh lines around his eyes and mouth suggested a sense of humor. But that was all we could ascertain. Did his smile contain gentleness? Was he a loving father? What made him jump out of bed in the morning? Whether he was a Mets fan, liked Bob Dylan, preferred mint chip ice cream, or could tell a joke was untraceable. What made Paul Paul was not on the silver anatomy table.

People are a collection of tissue, muscle, ligament, and bone—except, of course, they are not. The human equation never logically adds up. A breathing man's spark is infinitely more than his thirty trillion cells. Cellular collaboration extends far past the individual. Thirty trillion cells didn't paint the Sistine Chapel—Michelangelo did. You can say that Maya Angelou's poetry and Steve Jobs's iPhone came from their genius three-pound brains, but still, how did they manage to create something so beyond themselves? Microscopic cells and neural networks collaborate in a mind-boggling masterpiece of infinite activity happening every moment of every person's existence, outside of conscious awareness.

Science writer John Horgan has said neuroscience has a "Humpty Dumpty" problem. By the end of anatomy, my lab partners and I had broken down Paul's brain into bits, and all the world's biologists and all the world's neuroscientists couldn't put his eighty-six billion neurons back together again. Even if we could reassemble the dissected body, it wouldn't bring Paul back; every individual has a unique pattern shaped by his experiences. It's our daily interactions with the world that make us who we are and love that keeps us alive after our body is gone. Sixteen years later, I'd understand this firsthand.

In the midst of a January snowstorm, I went to see my mom's body one final time at the funeral home before it was cremated.

She'd died only four days before, and it had been just over two weeks since the night I got her strange text. Home from a long day on call in the ER as a weekend attending, I was curled up in bed watching the movie *Francis Ha* when I saw the message: "Hi kaellii I am home now ani An Ian not shut I will be comin g over tomorrow I will have to see how I feel lo b." My mom was a teacher and always a stickler for grammar, even in her texts. In one horrifying moment, I realized she was having a stroke.

Within hours of our arriving back at the hospital, my mom could no longer move, see, or talk, except for opening and closing her right hand. While she seemed to hear and understand us, she was locked in her own world. She and I developed a hand system to say "I love you." "I—*squeeze*—love—*squeeze*—you—*squeeze*." Three squeezes, back and forth, numerous times all throughout the day. While she could not speak, the distinct rhythm served as our sign that she was okay when we both knew everything was far from okay.

For nearly two weeks I sat fixed to her hospital bedside. My colleagues covered my patients as I experienced medicine from the other side. When my mom stopped returning the squeezes, I knew she was gone.

Life, as we all know, can change in an instant.

In the blur that followed, it was the love and kindness from friends, family, neighbors, coworkers, and even strangers that carried me through. A longtime friend, Anne Henry Maloney, unknowingly arrived at the hospital to be by my side moments before my mom took her last breath. Another dear friend, Carrie McKellogg, drove up from Washington, DC, taking time away from her high-powered government job and two young children to help us plan the funeral in the middle of an unusually cruel New York City winter. The task felt like organizing a shotgun wedding in a coma. In our grief, my family survived off the food baskets that arrived.

In the funeral home, despite the unexpectedly bright postmortem makeup, which would have made my mom chuckle, her face looked peaceful. Standing next to her body, I had the same familiar feeling I get with all the corpses I've seen—the body is there, but the person is gone. My mom's exuberant personality, melodic voice, and warm laugh echoed in my memory. *Where did all her energy go?* I wish I knew.

That night something strange happened.

My mom regularly watched my son Zay, who was a charming nearly-two-year-old at the time. They spent their days together reading books, playing games, and exploring the world. While he did not fully have the words to express it, Zay seemed painfully aware of his grandma's absence. He frequently asked for her. When we'd remind him that she got very sick, he'd announce, "Grandma's in my heart."

The day my mom was cremated, Zay began crying in the night. In the dark, my husband brought him to me, and I held my little boy close to my body. I felt comforted by his warmth and sweet smell. In his toddler drawl, he said a discernible "I love you," an unexpected and unprompted first. I beamed in the dark, hugging him tighter. Then he forcefully grabbed my hand. He gave me three distinct squeezes: one-*pause*-two-*pause*-three. The first squeeze I found surprising, the second one strange, and by the third one I was crying. Zay immediately fell asleep in my arms. I was suddenly wide awake.

Three squeezes to communicate "I love you" was the private language used between my mom and me. I had not shared this with my children or husband. Zay, while a deeply loving child, was never one to hold hands, except out of necessity. The evidence-based physician part of me thought this was surely a coincidence of a grieving mind looking for a sign. But as a human being sitting in the still night, it felt like a clear message of love from my mom saying, "Darling, please don't worry about me. I'm okay. I'm still with you."

I marvel at the enduring and mysterious bonds of love. The connections between us persist long after a person takes her final breath. We are emotionally and biologically linked through time in ways we don't fully understand. There is an old saying that you start medical school saying "I don't know" and leave saying "We don't know." I've dedicated my career to understanding life, yet I remain in awe of its mystery.

Acknowledgments

I am flooded with gratitude for the countless people who contributed in various ways to this book. From its inception, this project has been a labor of love, and I'm deeply thankful to all those who kindled the fire, lit the path, and traveled beside me on this adventure. As any author knows, it's a long journey from an idea to a book on the shelf. I'm awestruck how the spark of inspiration transforms into words on a page that then takes on a life of its own. In January 2014, as I sat for many long hours in my despair among the beeping at my mom's bedside in the Neuro ICU, I knew I could no longer ignore the growing call of the hidden factors of health and the story of the rabbits. I understood to truly transform health would require a broad audience far beyond the hospital walls and that I needed do my part to sound the alarm for change. I also knew I couldn't do it alone. I hope my story will inspire you to chase after some of your white rabbits too. The best part is all the wonderful people I've gotten to know along the way.

A huge heartfelt thank you to my superb publishing team at Simon & Schuster and Atria Books, which includes my marvelous editor, Sarah Pelz, for nurturing this manuscript and helping it take flight. You saw the beauty in the early idea and encouraged the story to develop intuitively, which was an incredible gift. Your thoughtful guidance, encouragement, and perspective made writing this book a great joy. Thank you also to Melanie Iglesias Pérez, Milena Brown, Felice Javit, Kyoko Watanabe, and the many others who helped tremendously along the way.

Acknowledgments

This book would not have been possible without the wonderful Dr. Maura Spiegel connecting me to Don Fehr, who is both an all-star literary agent and a lovely human being. Don, I greatly appreciate your kindness and endless persistence with various drafts of the proposal. I learned a tremendous amount with your guidance. It turns out the fifth draft is the charm!

A special thanks to the incredible Dedi Felman (aka the BookDoctor-West)—simply the best writing coach and collaborator an author could imagine! There is absolute magic when someone gets the essence of a project as it takes shape. Your wisdom, humor, logic, professionalism, compassion, and advice helped me stay on the road many times when I found myself veering toward enticing detours. Thank you for helping me navigate this first book to the finish with style. I grew both as a writer and a person throughout our adventure.

Another special note of thanks to Marjorie Korn, who closely read both early and late drafts of the manuscript. You are an inspiration as a writer, editor, and human being. I am so blessed to have had your thoughtful perspective, keen eagle eye, and fabulous sense of humor along with me on this journey. Your awesomeness astounds me! I'm also deeply indebted to my dear friends Dr. Sarah Heward and Marisa Plowden for encouraging me to pursue this project from the get-go and offering priceless feedback on countless iterations often right before looming deadlines. Thank you also to an amazing group of women who've had my back since college: Anne Maloney, Dana Sisitsky, Jen Wolosin, Lindsay Barnett, and Carrie McKellogg. You all give me strength beyond words and having you all to bounce ideas off and read sample drafts was priceless. I'm so glad we get to travel through life together.

This book is a tribute to so many wonderful patients I have encountered during my career. I hope I've done the spirit of your stories justice, albeit in disguise. It also builds on the generous work of so many experts across many fields. I am grateful to all whose work is featured. In addition, I wish to acknowledge the many clinicians, researchers, public health practitioners, students, mentors, and community leaders who have inspired me with their integrity, leadership, creativity, compassion, and time. A fraction of them include: Dr. Darrell Kirch (and the incredible staff at the Association of American Medical Colleges), Dr. Robert Nerem, Dr. Larry Guttmacher, Dr. Carola Eisenberg. Dr. John Hansen, Paula Smith, Ellen Caruso, Dr. Moshe Szyf, Dr. Paul Appelbaum, Dr. Lois Margaret Nora, Dr. Gary Belkin, Dr. Philip Alberti, Dr. Michael Sparer, Chelsea Clinton, Dr. Lisa Mellman, Dr. Ronald Reider, Dr. Myrna Weissman, Professor Richard Layard, Mark Williamson (and the staff at Action for Happiness), Dr. Natalie Gluck, Dr. Melissa Arbuckle, Cameron Schiller (and his lovely family), Dr. Christina Mangurian, Dr. Michael Devlin, Dr. Mary Sciutto, Dr. Harold Pincus, Dr. Ina Becker, Dr. David Strauss, Dr. Tim Walsh, Dr. Francis Levin, Dr. Allison Levin, Dr. Denzel Woode, Mary Anne Baldus, Lisa Colton, Helene Durham, Catherine O'Leary, Mary T. Coster, Margaret Gibson, Doris Pabon, Betzaida Rosado, Rosalyn Rodriguez, Juanita Wright, Evelyn Gantalao, Mary Ann A., Florence Leighton, Dr. Lucy Hunter, Dr. Nyota Pieh, Miguelina Espiritu, Elisandro De La Cruz, Fiona Woodman, Casey Pant, Boris Ingberg, Amnona Miller, Mary Devine, Dr. Fernando Taveres, Dr. Oren Messeri, Dr. Zeynep Altun, Dr. Mark Petrini, Dr. Brett Blatter, Dr. Renu Culas, Dr. Jack Pula, Dr. Kendra Campbell, Dr. Diana Samuel, Dr. Dianna Dragatsi, Dr. Zachary Freyberg, Wallis Post, Jessica Bowers, Elizabeth Grayer, Christy Turlington Burns (also Nan and Melissa at Every Mother Counts), Laura Talmus (at Beyond Differences), and Dr. Elizabeth Blackburn. In addition, I'd like to thank Dr. Reza Amighi and Dr. Tana-Grady Weliky, two wonderful mentors and colleagues who inspired the best in medicine. You are both dearly missed.

A debt of gratitude to Dr. Edward Hundert for instilling a fierce passion for medical professionalism from day one of my medical career and introducing me to Dr. Engel's lovely biopsychosocial model. The Ripple Effect is a tribute to your paradigm shifting vision of the concentric rings. A huge thank-you also to Dr. Brian Fallon and Dr. Arthur Barsky for your years of mentorship and supporting my intellectual curiosity about the mysterious link between physical and emotional symptoms. You both also encouraged me to write, for which I am eternally grateful. Dr. Janis Cutler (and Edith White) for supporting me over the years as I explored the national and international landscape of health care and medical education. Your work has inspired countless students to see the person behind the illness. Colman McCarthy, your gift of teaching peace is beyond words extraordinary. Your life's work is an inspiration to all. Thank you for being so generous with your time and spirit. The staff at Washington AIDS Partnership AmeriCorps Program led for the past twenty years by the phenomenal J. Channing Wickham. I am so honored to be among your distinguished alumni. The work you do creates endless ripples of compassion.

Speaking of compassion, I am intensely moved by the dedicated work that is done every day by frontline staff at New York-Presbyterian Hospital, Columbia University's Vagelos College of Physicians and Surgeons, Columbia's Mailman School of Public Health, as well as Mount Sinai Hospital, the University of Rochester School of Medicine, and Strong Memorial Hospital. I am grateful to have had academic homes at all of theses incredible places along with their affiliated hospitals over the past twenty years. I am inspired by their quest for continuous innovation and improvement.

A heartfelt thank-you to Dr. Marina Catallozzi at Columbia's Mailman School of Public Health, for nurturing my unorthodox initial project, and my advisor Dr. Mindy Thompson Fullilove for inspiring me in countless ways and helping me see the work through. Mindy, your ideas are changing the world for the better. Your lead and kind invitation to join the writing group made all the difference to transforming this dream into reality. Thank you to our amazing group in all its iterations (including Mindy, Maura, Ann Burack-Weiss, Jim Gilbert, Simon Fortin, John Kavanaugh, Craig Irvine, Jack Saul, Helena Hansen, and Priya Parker) for your feedback, encouragement, and guidance over the past several years. I feel so blessed. There is magic in those meetings.

In the spirit of the hidden factors, I don't believe *The Rabbit Effect* would have transformed from idea to words on a page without the community of The Writers Room, the urban sanctuary where I sit typing this line. Thank you to executive director Donna Brodie, the board of directors, and my fellow writers for providing the perfect blend of solitude, community, and inspiration. I'd also like to thank two extraordinary moms and storytellers, Tamara Jenkins and Sofia Coppola, for their writing tips along the way. You both are inspirations for me and countless others. A huge thanks also to Thom Blaylock, an incredible creative writer, thinker, and educator. Your writing workshop and enthusiasm kick-started this process. An extremely belated thank-you to my tenth-grade English teacher, Mrs. Anne-Marie Utter, at Reno High School. I have thought about your grammar lessons, which I severely undervalued at the time, on countless pages of this manuscript.

I'm also grateful to fellow physician writers including, Dr. Lloyd Sederer, Dr. Drew Ramsey, Dr. Jeffrey Lieberman, Dr. Rita Charon, Dr. David Forrest, Dr. Danielle Ofri, Dr. Pauline Chen, Dr. Deborah Cabanas, Dr. Jerome Groopman, Dr. Atul Gawande, Dr. Rachel Naomi Remen, Dr. Dean Ornish, Dr. Siddhartha Mukherjee, Dr. Deepak Chopra, Dr. Dan Siegel, and the late Dr. Oliver Sacks, Dr. Sherwin Nuland, and Dr. Richard Selzer. While some of you I know personally and others I know only through your stories and tidbits of advice, you've all paved the way. I have learned much through your lead and compassion. Thank you for all you do and inspire.

I am grateful for the support and encouragement of so many lovely friends who have listened to me talk about this project and encouraged it in many ways (some of you have read drafts) as it evolved over the years including: Dr. Amy Park, Dr. Karen Leitner, Dr. Lara Ford, Dr. Robert Berman, Dr. Jason Bauer, Dr. Ethan Ilzetski, Gabe Wolosin, Arlene Tschop, Pat and David Plowden, Dr. Greg Tau, Carl Ellis, Nicole Duncan, Sarah Traverso, Kitty Harding, Nan Nixon, Polly Flinch, Dr. David Schab, Ariel Kaminer, Dr. Diane McLean, Dr. Nicolas Oreskovic, Dr. Isabelle Chase, Roberta Benaman, Lisha Bai (and Sarah too!), Christine Lawry, Shelly Rossmeyer and Dean Pepe (and their lovely family), Joshua and Julia Gallu, Bess Oransky, Kristina Wels, Gary Kahn, Gitonga Kiara, Inosi Nyatta, Teresa Edleston, Jason Olim, Jason Rothstein, Marika Condos, Kerri Fersel-Bennet, Sara Kubersky, Francisca Villegas, Sarah Gaudreau, Laura MacDonald, Ken Geist, Walter and Jane Leppin (and their beautiful family), Dawn Burckley, Claire Cotter, Matt and Cary Bernstein, Catherine Del Guercio, Georgia Silvera Seamans, John Mcintosh, Kalia Doner, Dr. Eric Klinenberg, Dr. Caitlin Zaloom, Lorri Shackelford, Veronica Mainetti, Laurence Guguen, Lindsay McLean, Hadley Spanier, Cris Smith, Frank Van Riper, and Beverly Chen. There are many, many more.

And, of course, above all, I thank my wonderful family both by birth and marriage. I am blessed with a large extended family filled with amazing people I consider dear friends too. All have contributed in their way to my life and ideas for this book for which I am deeply thankful. In particular, I owe a debt of gratitude to my wonderful aunt and uncle, Drs. Deborah Harding and Victor Harding, for inspiring me to choose a career in medicine. You both sparked my curiosity and love of the field. My most wonderful dad, Bruce, thank you for your great sense of humor and encouraging my passion to pursue what I love throughout the years. Your unwavering support means the world. Mom, I know you are with me in spirit. And my superheroes: Padraic, the love of my life, and our most precious Max, Ryan, and Zay, I am eternally grateful for your enduring humor, patience, and compassion throughout the creation of this book. I couldn't have made it through all the late nights, early mornings, and long days of writing and rewriting without you all. The irony of describing the importance of relationships while I sequestered myself to complete the manuscript is not lost on me. I am eternally grateful how each of you brightens my days immeasurably with laughter and love.

Notes

INTRODUCTION

1 Kyle J. Foreman et al., "Forecasting Life Expectancy, Years of Life Lost, and All-Cause and Cause-Specific Mortality for 250 Causes of Death: Reference and Alternative Scenarios for 2016–40 for 195 Countries and Territories," *The Lancet* 392, no. 10159 (2018): 2052–90.

2 Anne Case and Angus Deaton, "Rising Morbidity and Mortality in Midlife Among White Non-Hispanic Americans in the 21st Century," *Proceedings of the National Academy of Sciences* 112, no. 49 (2015): 15078–83.

3 "Surviving the First Day: State of the World's Mothers," Save the Children Foundation, May 2013, https://www.savethechildren.org/content/dam/usa/reports/advocacy/sowm/sowm-2013.pdf; "The Issue," Every Mother Counts (accessed January 6, 2018), https://everymothercounts.org/our-story/the-issue/.

4 Nina Martin, Rene Montegue, "U.S. Has the Worst Rate of Maternal Deaths in the Developed World," NPR and ProPublica (May 12, 2017), https://www.npr.org/2017/05/12/528098789/u-s-has-the-worst-rate-of-maternal-deaths-in-the-developed-world; Nicholas J. Kassebaum et al., "Global, Regional, and National Levels of Maternal Mortality, 1990–2015: A Systematic Analysis for the Global Burden of Disease Study 2015," *The Lancet* 388, no. 10053 (2016): 1775–1812; "Maternal Health in the United States," Maternal Health Task Force at the Harvard Chan School Center of Excellence in Maternal and Child Health (accessed January 16, 2019), https://www.mhtf.org/topics/maternal-health-in-the-united-states/.

5 Selena Gonzales and Bradley Sawyer, "How Do Mortality Rates in the U.S. Compare to Other Countries?" Kaiser Family Foundation (May 22, 2017), https://www.healthsystemtracker.org/chart-collection/mortality-rates-u-s-compare-countries/?_sft_category=health-well-being#item-start; for ongoing updates, check "Health System Dashboard," Peterson-Kaiser Health System Tracker (accessed January 15, 2019), https://www.healthsystemtracker.org/dashboard/.

6 Joachim O. Hero, Alan M. Zaslavsky, and Robert J. Blendon, "The United States Leads Other Nations in Differences by Income in Perceptions of Health and Health Care," *Health Affairs* 36, no. 6 (2017): 1032–40.

7   Richard G. Wilkinson and Kate E. Pickett, "Income Inequality and Social Dys-
     function," *Annual Review of Sociology* 35 (2009): 493–511; Richard E. Wilkinson
     and Kate E. Pickett, "Income Inequality and Health: A Causal Review," Agency
     for Healthcare Research and Quality, Rockville, MD (reviewed July 2015), http://
     www.ahrq.gov/professionals/education/curriculum-tools/population-health/pickett
     .html; Richard Wilkinson, "How Economic Inequality Harms Society," filmed July 2011
     at TEDGlobal, video, 3:02, https://www.ted.com/talks/richard_wilkinson?language
     =en#t-178485

8   Kate E. Pickett and Richard G. Wilkinson, "Child Well-Being and Income Inequality
     in Rich Societies: Ecological Cross Sectional Study," *BMJ* 335, no. 7629 (2007): 1080.

9   James Banks et al., "Disease and Disadvantage in the United States and in England,"
     JAMA 295, no. 17 (2006): 2037–45.

10   OECD health data (2017), Health at a Glance. Paris: Organisation for Economic
     Co-operation and Development, http://www.oecd.org/health/health-systems/Health
     -Spending-Latest-Trends-Brief.pdf.

11   Liz Hamel et al., "The Burden of Medical Debt: Results from the Kaiser Family
     Foundation," *New York Times* medical bills survey (2016).

12   Darrell Kirch, president and CEO of the Association of American Medical Colleges,
     in discussion with the author (February 2018).

13   Centers for Medicare & Medicaid Services, Office of the Actuary, National Health
     Statistics Group, "The Nation's Health Dollar ($3.5 Trillion), Calendar Year
     2017, Where It Went," https://www.cms.gov/Research-Statistics-Data-and-Systems
     /Statistics-Trends-and-Reports/NationalHealthExpendData/Downloads/PieChart
     SourcesExpenditures.pdf.

14   Zac Auter, "U.S. Uninsured Rate Steady at 12.2% in Fourth Quarter of 2017," Gallup
     (January 16, 2018), https://news.gallup.com/poll/225383/uninsured-rate-steady
     -fourth-quarter-2017.aspx.

15   "Health Spending and the Economy," Health System Dashboard, Peterson-Kaiser
     Health System Tracker (accessed December 6, 2018), https://www.healthsystem
     tracker.org/dashboard/.

16   J. Michael McGinnis et al., "The Case for More Active Policy Attention to Health
     Promotion," *Health Affairs* 21, no. 2 (2002): 78–93; Steven A. Schroeder, "We Can
     Do Better—Improving the Health of the American People," *New England Journal of
     Medicine* 357, no. 12 (2007): 1221–28.

17   John B. McKinlay and Sonja M. McKinlay, "The Questionable Contribution of
     Medical Measures to the Decline of Mortality in the United States in the Twentieth
     Century," *The Milbank Quarterly* 55, no. 3 (1977): 405–28.

18   Robert Nerem, professor emeritus and Parker H. Petit distinguished chair for engi-
     neering in medicine, Georgia Institute of Technology, in discussion with the author
     (February 2017), https://petitinstitute.gatech.edu/robert-nerem.

19   Robert M. Nerem, Murina J. Levesque, and J. Fredrick Cornhill, "Social Environ-
     ment as a Factor in Diet-Induced Atherosclerosis," *Science* 208, no. 4451 (1980):
     1475–76.

Notes

CHAPTER ONE

1 George L. Engel, "The Need for a New Medical Model: A Challenge for Biomedicine," *Science* 196, no. 4286 (1977): 129–36.
2 J. Michael McGinnis, Pamela Williams-Russo, and James R. Knickman, "The Case for More Active Policy Attention to Health Promotion," *Health Affairs* 21, no. 2 (2002): 78–93.
3 Bruce G. Link and Jo Phelan, "Social Conditions as Fundamental Causes of Disease," *Journal of Health and Social Behavior* (1995): 80–94.
4 Mary Shaw, Richard Mitchell, and Danny Dorling, "Time for a Smoke? One Cigarette Reduces Your Life by 11 Minutes," *BMJ* 320, no. 7226 (2000): 53.

CHAPTER TWO

1 Colin Freeman, "How a Farewell Cuddle Revived a Dying Baby," *The Telegraph* (March 13, 2015), https://www.telegraph.co.uk/news/worldnews/australiaandthe pacific/australia/11471307/How-a-farewell-cuddle-revived-a-dying-baby.html.
2 Michael Inbar, "Mom's Hug Revives Baby That Was Pronounced Dead," *Today* (October 14, 2016), https://www.today.com/parents/moms-hug-revives-baby-was -pronounced-dead-2D80554298.
3 Brie Schwards, "Her Baby Was Pronounced Dead at Birth, But When This Mother Held Her Tiny Son, a Miracle Happened," *Redbook* (March 11, 2015).
4 Moshe Szyf, epigenetic researcher/pioneer, James McGill Professorship and GlaxoSmithKline-CIHR Chair in Pharmacology at McGill University, in discussion with the author (November 2017).
5 Ian C. G. Weaver et al., "Epigenetic Programming by Maternal Behavior," *Nature Neuroscience* 7, no. 8 (2004): 847; Michael J. Meaney and Moshe Szyf, "Environmental Programming of Stress Responses Through DNA Methylation: Life at the Interface Between a Dynamic Environment and a Fixed Genome," *Dialogues in Clinical Neuroscience* 7, no. 2 (2005): 103.
6 L. H. Lumey et al., "Cohort Profile: The Dutch Hunger Winter Families Study," *International Journal of Epidemiology* 36, no. 6 (2007): 1196–1204.
7 Peter Ekamper et al., "Independent and Additive Association of Prenatal Famine Exposure and Intermediary Life Conditions With Adult Mortality Between Age 18–63 Years," *Social Science & Medicine* 119 (2014): 232–9.
8 Jessica L. Saben et al., "Maternal Metabolic Syndrome Programs Mitochondrial Dysfunction Via Germline Changes Across Three Generations," *Cell Reports* 16, no. 1 (2016): 1–8.
9 Daniel A. Notterman and Colter Mitchell, "Epigenetics and Understanding the Impact of Social Determinants of Health," *Pediatric Clinics* 62, no. 5 (2015): 1227–40.
10 Haoyang Lu et al., "DNA Methylation: A Hand Behind Neurodegenerative Diseases," *Frontiers in Aging Neuroscience* 5 (2013): 85.
11 Marilla Steuter-Martin and Loreen Pindera, "Looking Back on the 1998 Ice Storm 20 Years Later," CBS News (January 4, 2018), https://www.cbc.ca/news/canada /montreal/ice-storm-1998-1.4469977.
12 Moshe Szyf, "How Early Life Experience Is Written into DNA," filmed July 2016

at TEDx Bratislava, Bratislava, Slovakia, video, 16:36, https://www.ted.com/talks/moshe_szyf_how_early_life_experience_is_written_into_dna.

13 David P. Laplante et al., "Project Ice Storm: Prenatal Maternal Stress Affects Cognitive and Linguistic Functioning in 5½-Year-Old Children," *Journal of the American Academy of Child & Adolescent Psychiatry* 47, no. 9 (2008): 1063–72.

14 Lei Cao-Lei et al., "DNA Methylation Signatures Triggered by Prenatal Maternal Stress Exposure to a Natural Disaster: Project Ice Storm," *PLOS ONE* 9, no. 9 (2014): e107653.

15 _____. "DNA Methylation Mediates the Effect of Exposure to Prenatal Maternal Stress on Cytokine Production in Children at Age 13½ Years: Project Ice Storm," *Clinical Epigenetics* 8, no. 1 (2016): 54.

16 Mary S. Ainsworth and John Bowlby, "An Ethological Approach to Personality Development," *American Psychologist* 46, no. 4 (1991): 333; Inge Bretherton, "The Origins of Attachment Theory: John Bowlby and Mary Ainsworth," *Developmental Psychology* 28, no. 5 (1992): 759.

17 Marinus H. Van Ijzendoorn and Pieter M. Kroonenberg, "Cross-Cultural Patterns of Attachment: A Meta-Analysis of the Strange Situation," *Child Development* (1988): 147–56.

18 Markus Quirin et al., "Adult Attachment Insecurity and Hippocampal Cell Density," *Social Cognitive and Affective Neuroscience* 5, no. 1 (2009): 39-47; Pascal Vrticka and Patrik Vuilleumier, "Neuroscience of Human Social Interactions and Adult Attachment Style," *Frontiers in Human Neuroscience* 6 (2012): 212; Mario Mikulincer and Philip R. Shaver, "An Attachment Perspective on Psychopathology," *World Psychiatry* 11, no. 1 (2012): 11–5; Jennifer Puig et al., "Predicting Adult Physical Illness From Infant Attachment: A Prospective Longitudinal Study," *Health Psychology* 32, no. 4 (2013): 409.

19 Liz Mineo, "Good Genes Are Nice, But Joy Is Better," *The Harvard Gazette* (April 11, 2017), https://news.harvard.edu/gazette/story/2017/04/over-nearly-80-years-harvard-study-has-been-showing-how-to-live-a-healthy-and-happy-life/.

20 George Vaillant, "Yes I Stand by My Words, 'Happiness Equals Love—Full Stop,'" *Positive Psychology News* (July 16, 2009), https://positivepsychologynews.com/news/george-vaillant/200907163163; Joshua Wolf Shenk, "What Makes Us Happy?" *The Atlantic* (June 2009), https://www.theatlantic.com/magazine/archive/2009/06/what-makes-us-happy/307439/.

21 Nathalie Charpak, Juan G. Ruiz-Peláez, and Yves Charpak, "Rey-Martinez Kangaroo Mother Program: An Alternative Way of Caring for Low Birth Weight Infants? One Year Mortality in a Two Cohort Study," *Pediatrics* 94, no. 6 (1994): 804–10.

22 Lena Corner, "Saving Babies' Lives by Carrying Them Like Kangaroos," *The Atlantic* (February 7, 2017), https://www.theatlantic.com/health/archive/2017/02/kangaroo-care/515844/.

23 Ellen O. Boundy et al., "Kangaroo Mother Care and Neonatal Outcomes: A Meta-Analysis," *Pediatrics* 137, no. 1 (2016): e20152238.

24 Paul J. Zak, Angela A. Stanton, and Sheila Ahmadi, "Oxytocin Increases Generosity in Humans," *PLOS ONE* 2, no. 11 (2007): e1128.

25 Robin I. M. Dunbar, "The Social Role of Touch in Humans and Primates: Behavioural Function and Neurobiological Mechanisms," *Neuroscience & Biobehavioral Reviews* 34, no. 2 (2010): 260–8; Susan Paulson, "'Beauty Is More than Skin Deep,' An Ethnographic Study of Beauty Therapists and Older Women," *Journal of*

Aging Studies 22, no. 3 (2008): 256–65; *Daily Mail Reporter*, "The Ladies Who Hang on to Hairdressers Longer than Husbands: Average Woman Keeps Same Stylist for More Than 12 Years, While Marriage Lasts 11," *Daily Mail* (November 11, 2013), https://www.dailymail.co.uk/femail/article-2502231/The-ladies-hang-hairdressers -longer-husbands.html.

26 Abraham Verghese and Ralph I. Horwitz, "In Praise of the Physical Examination," *BMJ* 339 (2009): b5448.

27 Karen M. Grewen et al., "Warm Partner Contact Is Related to Lower Cardiovascular Reactivity," *Behavioral Medicine* 29, no. 3 (2003): 123–30; Alberto Gallace and Charles Spence, "The Science of Interpersonal Touch: An Overview," *Neuroscience & Biobehavioral Reviews* 34, no. 2 (2010): 246–59.

28 Alexandra Zaslow, "Sonogram Shows Dying Twin Holding His Sister's Hand in the Womb," *Today* (February 18, 2016), https://www.today.com/parents/sonogram -shows-dying-twin-holding-his-sister-s-hand-womb-t74416.

29 James A. Coan, Hillary S. Schaefer, and Richard J. Davidson, "Lending a Hand: Social Regulation of the Neural Response to Threat," *Psychological Science* 17, no. 12 (2006): 1032–39.

30 Pavel Goldstein et al., "Brain-to-Brain Coupling During Handholding Is Associated with Pain Reduction," *Proceedings of the National Academy of Sciences* 115, no. 11 (2018): e2528–e2537.

31 Frank E. Hanson et al., "Synchrony and Flash Entrainment in a New Guinea Firefly," *Science* 174, no. 4005 (1971): 161–4.

32 Alejandro Pérez, Manuel Carreiras, and Jon Andoni Duñabeitia, "Brain-to-Brain Entrainment: EEG Interbrain Synchronization While Speaking and Listening," *Scientific Reports* 7, no. 1 (2017): 4190.

33 Tiffany Field, "Massage Therapy Research Review," *Complementary Therapies in Clinical Practice* 24 (2016): 19–31.

34 Tiffany Field. *Touch* (Massachusetts: MIT Press, 2014).

35 Sayuri M. Naruse, Piers L. Cornelissen, and Mark Moss, "To Give Is Better than to Receive? Couples Massage Significantly Benefits Both Partners' Well-Being," *Journal of Health Psychology* (2018), https://doi.org/10.1177/1359105318763502.

36 Sheldon Cohen et al., "Does Hugging Provide Stress-Buffering Social Support? A Study of Susceptibility to Upper Respiratory Infection and Illness," *Psychological Science* 26, no. 2 (2015): 135–47.

37 Karen M. Grewen et al., "Warm Partner Contact Cs Related to Lower Cardiovascular Reactivity," *Behavioral Medicine* 29, no. 3 (2003): 123–30.

38 Eliska Prochazkova and Mariska E. Kret, "Connecting Minds and Sharing Emotions Through Mimicry: A Neurocognitive Model of Emotional Contagion," *Neuroscience & Biobehavioral Reviews* 80 (2017): 99–114.

39 George Szekeres, "Professor George Szekeres (1911-2005), Mathematician," interview by Imogen Jubb (2004), https://www.science.org.au/learning/general-audience /history/interviews-australian-scientists/professor-george-szekeres-1911#4.

40 Lillian Saleh, "True Love's Lasting Testament," news.com.au (August 31, 2005); Jamie Morgan, "Together Forever: One Couple's 69-Year Love Story," *The Advertiser* (August 31, 2005).

41 Jody Heymann, Amy Raub, and Alison Earle, "Creating and Using New Data Sources to Analyze the Relationship Between Social Policy and Global Health: The Case of Maternal Leave," *Public Health Reports* 126, suppl. 3 (2011): 127–34.

Notes

CHAPTER THREE

1   Clarke Stout et al., "Unusually Low Incidence of Death From Myocardial Infarction: Study of an Italian American Community in Pennsylvania," *JAMA* 188, no. 10 (1964): 845–9; John Bruhn and Stewart Wolf. *The Roseto Story: An Anatomy of Health* (University of Oklahoma Press, 2013). Malcolm Gladwell, *Outliers: The Story of Success* (UK: Hachette, 2008).

2   Robert D. Putnam, *Bowling Alone: The Collapse and Revival of American Community* (New York: Simon & Schuster, 2001).

3   Brenda Egolf et al., "The Roseto Effect: A 50-Year Comparison of Mortality Rates," *American Journal of Public Health* 82, no. 8 (1992): 1089–92.

4   Emiko Jozuka, "In the Land of the Immortals: Japan's Centenarian Pop Band," *CNN* (June 22, 2018), https://www.cnn.com/2018/06/08/health/japan-longevity-centenarians-aging-population/index.html.

5   G. Oscar Anderson, Colette Thayer, AARP Research, "Loneliness and Social Connections: A National Survey of Adults 45 and Older," *AARP* (September 2018), https://www.aarp.org/research/topics/life/info-2018/loneliness-social-connections.html?CMP=RDRCT-PRI-HOMFAM-073118; Knowledge Networks and Insight Policy Research, "Loneliness Among Older Adults: A National Survey of Adults 45 and Older," AARP (September 2010), https://assets.aarp.org/rgcenter/general/loneliness_2010.pdf; "Cigna 2018 U.S. loneliness index" (accessed January 12, 2019), https://www.cigna.com/assets/docs/newsroom/loneliness-survey-2018-fact-sheet.pdf.

6   Carla M. Perissinotto, Irena Stijacic Cenzer, and Kenneth E. Covinsky, "Loneliness in Older Persons: A Predictor of Functional Decline and Death," *Archives of Internal Medicine* 172, no. 14 (2012): 1078–84.

7   Susan Davidson and Phil Rossall, "Evidence Review: Loneliness in Later Life," *ageUK* (updated July 2015), https://www.ageuk.org.uk/globalassets/age-uk/documents/reports-and-publications/reports-and-briefings/health—wellbeing/rb_june15_lonelines_in_later_life_evidence_review.pdf.

8   G. Berguno et al., "Children's Experience of Loneliness at School and Its Relation to Bullying and the Quality of Teacher Interventions," *The Qualitative Report* 9, no. 3 (2004): 483–499. Retrieved from http://nsuworks.nova.edu/tqr/vol9/iss3/7.

9   Brett V. Brown, ed. *Key Indicators of Child and Youth Well-Being: Completing the Picture.* Psychology Press, 2008, https://books.google.com/books?id=vwp8dDedy-cC&pg=PT244&lpg=PT244&dq=#v=onepage&q&f=false.

10   John Cacioppo, "Epidemic of Loneliness," *Psychology Today* (May 3, 2009), https://www.psychologytoday.com/us/blog/connections/200905/epidemic-loneliness).

11   Cameron Crowe, "So Lonely I Could Cry," *The Guardian* (January 10, 2002), "http://www.theguardian.com/film/2002/jan/11/artsfeatures2.

12   Julianne Holt-Lunstad, Wendy Birmingham, and Brandon Q. Jones, "Is There Something Unique About Marriage? The Relative Impact of Marital Status, Relationship Quality, and Network Social Support on Ambulatory Blood Pressure and Mental Health," *Annals of Behavioral Medicine* 35, no. 2 (2008): 239–44; Julianne Holt-Lunstad, Wendy C. Birmingham, and Kathleen C. Light, "Relationship Quality and Oxytocin: Influence of Stable and Modifiable Aspects of Relationships," *Journal of Social and Personal Relationships* 32, no. 4 (2015): 472–90.

13   Carla M. Perissinotto, Irena Stijacic Cenzer, and Kenneth E. Covinsky, "Loneliness

in Older Persons: A Predictor of Functional Decline and Death," *Archives of Internal Medicine* 172, no. 14 (2012): 1078–84.

14 Julianne Holt-Lunstad, "So Lonely I Could Die," American Psychological Association, Session 3328 (August 5, 2017), https://www.apa.org/news/press/releases /2017/08/lonely-die.aspx; Partha Das, "Study Unveils Loneliness Increases the Risk of Early Death, More Deadlier Compared to Obesity," *The Science Times* (August 7, 2017), http://www.sciencetimes.com/articles/17720/20170807/study-unveils -loneliness-increases-risk-early-death-more-deadlier-obesity.htm.

15 Nicole K. Valtorta et al., "Loneliness and Social Isolation as Risk Factors for Coronary Heart Disease and Stroke: Systematic Review and Meta-Analysis of Longitudinal Observational Studies," *Heart* 102, no. 13 (2016): 1009–16.

16 Julianne Holt-Lunstad et al., "Loneliness and Social Isolation as Risk Factors for Mortality: A Meta-Analytic Review," *Perspectives on Psychological Science* 10, no. 2 (2015): 227–37.

17 Naomi I. Eisenberger, Matthew D. Lieberman, and Kipling D. Williams, "Does Rejection Hurt? An fMRI Study of Social Exclusion," *Science* 302, no. 5643 (2003): 290–92.

18 Ethan Kross et al., "Social Rejection Shares Somatosensory Representations with Physical Pain," *Proceedings of the National Academy of Sciences* 108, no. 15 (2011): 6270–75.

19 Teemu Ryymin, "Tuberculosis-Threatened Children: The Rise and Fall of a Medical Concept in Norway, c. 1900–1960," *Medical History* 52, no. 3 (2008): 347–64.

20 Sheldon Cohen et al., "Social Ties and Susceptibility to the Common Cold," *JAMA* 277, no. 24 (1997): 1940–44.

21 René A. Spitz, "Hospitalism: An Inquiry into the Genesis of Psychiatric Conditions in Early Childhood," *The Psychoanalytic Study of the Child* 1, no. 1 (1945): 53–74.

22 "The Devastating Effects of Isolation on Social Behaviour," *The Brain*, McGill University (accessed January 13, 2019), http://thebrain.mcgill.ca/flash/capsules/histoire _bleu06.html.

23 René A. Spitz and Katherine M. Wolf, "Anaclitic Depression: An Inquiry into the Genesis of Psychiatric Conditions in Early Childhood II," *The Psychoanalytic Study of the Child* 2, no. 1 (1946): 313–42; René A. Spitz, "The Role of Ecological Factors in Emotional Development in Infancy," *Child Development* (1949): 145–55.

24 Charles A. Nelson et al., "Cognitive Recovery in Socially Deprived Young Children: The Bucharest Early Intervention Project," *Science* 318, no. 5858 (2007): 1937–40.

25 Ibid.

26 Avshalom Caspi et al., "Socially Isolated Children 20 Years Later: Risk of Cardiovascular Disease," *Archives of Pediatrics & Adolescent Medicine* 160, no. 8 (2006): 805–11.

27 Andrea Danese et al., "Adverse Childhood Experiences and Adult Risk Factors for Age-Related Disease: Depression, Inflammation, and Clustering of Metabolic Risk Markers," *Archives of Pediatrics & Adolescent Medicine* 163, no. 12 (2009): 1135–43.

28 Russell A. Hill and Robin I. M. Dunbar, "Social Network Size in Humans," *Human Nature* 14, no. 1 (2003): 53–72.

29 John T. Cacioppo et al., "Do Lonely Days Invade the Nights? Potential Social Modulation of Sleep Efficiency," *Psychological Science* 3, no. 4 (2002): 384–87.

30   Louise C. Hawkley et al., "Loneliness Is a Unique Predictor of Age-Related Differences in Systolic Blood Pressure," *Psychology and Aging* 21, no. 1 (2006): 152; Steve W. Cole et al., "Social Regulation of Gene Expression in Human Leukocytes," *Genome Biology* 8, no. 9 (2007): R189.

31   Sally S. Dickerson and Margaret E. Kemeny, "Acute Stressors and Cortisol Responses: A Theoretical Integration and Synthesis of Laboratory Research," *Psychological Bulletin* 130, no. 3 (2004): 355.

32   James S. House, Karl R. Landis, and Debra Umberson, "Social Relationships and Health," *Science* 241, no. 4865 (1988): 540–45.

33   Julianne Holt-Lunstad, Timothy B. Smith, and J. Bradley Layton, "Social Relationships and Mortality Risk: A Meta-Analytic Review," *PLOS Medicine* 7, no. 7 (2010): e1000316.

34   Sheldon Cohen et al., "Social Ties and Susceptibility to the Common Cold," *JAMA* 277, no. 24 (1997): 1940–44.

35   Debra Umberson and Jennifer Karas Montez, "Social Relationships and Health: A Flashpoint for Health Policy," *Journal of Health and Social Behavior* 51, no. 1, suppl. (2010): S54–S66.

36   Sarah D. Pressman et al., "Loneliness, Social Network Size, and Immune Response to Influenza Vaccination in College Freshmen," *Health Psychology* 24, no. 3 (2005): 297.

37   Caroline E. Jenkinson et al., "Is Volunteering a Public Health Intervention? A Systematic Review and Meta-Analysis of the Health and Survival of Volunteers," *BMC Public Health* 13, no. 1 (2013): 773.

38   Kay Cassill, "Stress Has Hit Roseto, Pa., Once the Town Heart Disease Passed By" (June 16, 1980), http://people.com/archive/stress-has-hit-roseto-pa-once-the-town-heart-disease-passed-by-vol-13-no-24/.

39   Nicholas A. Christakis and James H. Fowler, "The Spread of Obesity in a Large Social Network Over 32 Years," *New England Journal of Medicine* 357, no. 4 (2007): 370–79.

40   _____. "The Collective Dynamics of Smoking in a Large Social Network," *New England Journal of Medicine* 358, no. 21 (2008): 2249–58.

41   _____. "Friendship and Natural Selection," *Proceedings of the National Academy of Sciences* 111, suppl. 3 (2014): 10796–801.

42   Suma Jacob et al., "Paternally Inherited HLA Alleles Are Associated With Women's Choice of Male Odor," *Nature Genetics* 30, no. 2 (2002): 175.

43   Crista N. Crittenden et al., "Social Integration and Pulmonary Function in the Elderly," *Health Psychology* 33, no. 6 (2014): 535.

44   Bryan D. James et al., "Late-Life Social Activity and Cognitive Decline in Old Age," *Journal of the International Neuropsychological Society* 17, no. 6 (2011): 998–1005.

45   Lauren Gallagher, "Garrett Sathre Brings Pop-Up Picnic to Life in San Francisco," *The Examiner* (October 11, 2011), https://archives.sfexaminer.com/sanfrancisco/garrett-sathre-brings-pop-up-picnic-to-life-in-san-francisco/Content?oid=2183342.

46   Carla Marinucci, "Lili Smith, 15, Dies: Activist with Disability" (October 16, 2009), https://www.sfgate.com/bayarea/article/Lili-Smith-15-dies-activist-with-disability-3283889.php; "Our Inspiration: Lili Rachel Smith," Beyond Differences (accessed January 24, 2019).

47   "Beyond Differences," (accessed January 24, 2019), https://www.beyonddifferences.org/.

48 "No One Eats Alone" (accessed January 24, 2019), https://www.nooneeatsalone.org/.

49 Laura Talmus, cofounder and executive director of Beyond Differences in conversation with the author, January 24, 2019.

50 Karen Allen, Jim Blascovich, and Wendy B. Mendes, "Cardiovascular Reactivity and the Presence of Pets, Friends, and Spouses: The Truth About Cats and Dogs," *Psychosomatic Medicine* 64, no. 5 (2002): 727–39.

51 Mwenya Mubanga et al., "Dog Ownership and the Risk of Cardiovascular Disease and Death–A Nationwide Cohort Study," *Scientific Reports* 7, no. 1 (2017): 15821.

52 "New BarkBox Study Finds Dogs Make People Better, Happier and Healthier Humans," *Bark* (accessed December 10, 2018), https://bark.co/barkgoodpartners/new-barkbox-study-finds-dogs-make-people-better-happier-and-healthier-humans/.

53 Emma Elsworthy, "Over a Third of People Prefer Their Pets to Their Partner, Study Finds," *The Independent* (February 1, 2018), https://www.independent.co.uk/property/house-and-home/pets/pets-partners-preference-cats-dogs-kittens-puppies-survey-research-a8188866.html.

CHAPTER FOUR

1 David Sturt and Todd Nordstrom, "10 Shocking Workplace Stats You Need to Know," *Forbes* (March 8, 2018), https://www.forbes.com/sites/davidsturt/2018/03/08/10-shocking-workplace-stats-you-need-to-know/#39a6f116f3af.

2 Steven Sauter et al., "Stress at Work," *DHHS (NIOSH) Publication* 99–101 (1999): 1–25.

3 "The General Social Survey," NORC at the University of Chicago (accessed January 13, 2019), http://gss.norc.org/; Emma Seppälä and Marissa King, "Burnout at Work Isn't Just About Exhaustion. It's Also About Loneliness, " *Harvard Business Review* (June 29, 2017), https://hbr.org/2017/06/burnout-at-work-isnt-just-about-exhaustion-its-also-about-loneliness.

4 Wilmar B. Schaufeli, Michael P. Leiter, and Christina Maslach, "Burnout: 35 Years of Research and Practice," *Career Development International* 14, no. 3 (2009): 204–20.

5 Siang Yong Tan and A. Yip, "Hans Selye (1907–1982): Founder of the Stress Theory," *Singapore Medical Journal* 59, no. 4 (2018): 170.

6 Robert Frost, "A Servant to Servants," *North of Boston*. New York: Henry Holt and Co., 1915.

7 Hans Selye, "A Syndrome Produced by Diverse Nocuous Agents," *Nature* 138, no. 3479 (1936): 32.

8 Bruce S. McEwen, "Protective and Damaging Effects of Stress Mediators," *New England Journal of Medicine* 338, no. 3 (1998): 171–9; Richard Schulz and Scott R. Beach, "Caregiving as a Risk Factor for Mortality: The Caregiver Health Effects Study," *JAMA* 282, no. 23 (1999): 2215–19; Jos F. Brosschot, William Gerin, and Julian F. Thayer, "The Perseverative Cognition Hypothesis: A Review of Worry, Prolonged Stress-Related Physiological Activation, and Health," *Journal of Psychosomatic Research* 60, no. 2 (2006): 113–24.

9 Clare L. Stacey, "Finding Dignity in Dirty Work: The Constraints and Rewards of Low Wage Home Care Labour," *Sociology of Health & Illness* 27, no. 6 (2005): 831–54.

Notes

10 Michael Marmot, "Redefining Public Health: Epidemiology and Social Stratification," interview with Harry Kreisler, Institute of International Studies, UC Berkeley (March 18, 2002), http://globetrotter.berkeley.edu/people2/Marmot/marmot-con4.html.

11 Michael G. Marmot et al., "Employment Grade and Coronary Heart Disease in British Civil Servants," *Journal of Epidemiology & Community Health* 32, no. 4 (1978): 244–49.

12 _____. "Health Inequalities Among British Civil Servants: The Whitehall II Study," *The Lancet* 337, no. 8754 (1991): 1387–93.

13 _____. "Redefining Public Health: Epidemiology and Social Stratification," interview with Harry Kreisler, Institute of International Studies, UC Berkeley (March 18, 2002), http://globetrotter.berkeley.edu/people2/Marmot/marmot-con3.html.

14 Stephen A. Stansfeld et al., "Work Characteristics Predict Psychiatric Disorder: Prospective Results from the Whitehall II Study," *Occupational and Environmental Medicine* 56, no. 5 (1999): 302–7.

15 Sunday Azagba and Mesbah F. Sharaf, "Psychosocial Working Conditions and the Utilization of Health-care Services," *BMC Public Health* 11, no. 1 (2011): 642.

16 Monique Valcour, "The Power of Dignity in the Workplace," *Harvard Business Review* (April 28, 2014), https://hbr.org/2014/04/the-power-of-dignity-in-the-workplace.

17 Christine Porath, "Half of Employees Don't Feel Respected by Their Bosses," *Harvard Business Review* (November 9, 2014), https://hbr.org/2014/11/half-of-employees-dont-feel-respected-by-their-bosses; Tony Schwartz and Christine Porath, "The Power of Meeting Your Employees' Needs," *Harvard Business Review* 26, no. 6 (2014): 442–57.

18 John F. Helliwell et al., *Happiness at Different Ages: The Social Context Matters*, no. w25121, National Bureau of Economic Research (2018), https://www.nber.org/papers/w25121.

19 Ed Diener and Micaela Y. Chan, "Happy People Live Longer: Subjective Well-Being Contributes to Health and Longevity," *Applied Psychology: Health and Well-Being* 3, no. 1 (2011): 1–43.

20 Mihaly Csikszentmihalyi and Judith LeFevre, "Optimal Experience in Work and Leisure," *Journal of Personality and Social Psychology* 56, no. 5 (1989): 815.

21 Matthew A. Killingsworth and Daniel T. Gilbert, "A Wandering Mind Is an Unhappy Mind," *Science* 330, no. 6006 (2010): 932.

22 Schwartz and Porath, "The Power of Meeting Your Employees' Needs."

23 Androniki Naska et al., "Siesta in Healthy Adults and Coronary Mortality in the General Population," *Archives of Internal Medicine* 167, no. 3 (2007): 296–301.

24 Kyle J. Foreman et al., "Forecasting Life Expectancy, Years of Life Lost, and All-Cause and Cause-Specific Mortality for 250 Causes of Death: Reference and Alternative Scenarios for 2016–40 for 195 Countries and Territories," *The Lancet* 392, no. 10159 (2018): 2052–90.

25 Daniel R. Witte et al., "A Meta-Analysis of Excess Cardiac Mortality on Monday," *European Journal of Epidemiology* 20, no. 5 (2005): 401–6.

26 For information on starting your own workplace walking group, see the American Heart Association's Workplace Walking Program Kit, available at http://www.heart.org/HEARTORG/HealthyLiving/WorkplaceHealth/EmployerResources/The-American-Heart-Associations-Workplace-Walking-Program-Kit_UCM_460433_Article.jsp#.Wvz1qC_Mx-U.

Notes

27 William Burnett and David John Evans, *Designing Your Life: How to Build a Well-Lived, Joyful Life* (New York: Knopf, 2016).

28 Amy Poehler, *Yes Please* (New York: HarperCollins, 2014).

29 James H. Fowler and Nicholas A. Christakis, "Dynamic Spread of Happiness in a Large Social Network: Longitudinal Analysis Over 20 Years in the Framingham Heart Study," *BMJ* 337 (2008): a2338.

30 Steven H. Woolf, "How Are Income and Wealth Linked to Health and Longevity?" (2015), https://www.urban.org/sites/default/files/publication/49116/2000178-How-are-Income-and-Wealth-Linked-to-Health-and-Longevity.pdf.

31 Joachim O. Hero, Alan M. Zaslavsky, and Robert J. Blendon, "The United States Leads Other Nations in Differences by Income in Perceptions of Health and Health Care," *Health Affairs* 36, no. 6 (2017): 1032–40.

32 Andrew T. Jebb et al., "Happiness, Income Satiation and Turning Points Around the World," *Nature Human Behaviour* 2, no. 1 (2018): 33.

33 Daniel Kahneman and Angus Deaton, "High Income Improves Evaluation of Life But Not Emotional Well-Being," *Proceedings of the National Academy of Sciences* 107, no. 38 (2010): 16489–93.

34 Joachim O. Hero, Alan M. Zaslavsky, and Robert J. Blendon, "The United States Leads Other Nations in Differences by Income in Perceptions of Health and Health Care," *Health Affairs* 36, no. 6 (2017): 1032–40.

35 Oxfam, "Reward Work, Not Wealth," *Oxfam Briefing Paper* (2018).

36 "Mo Gawdat's Moonshot for Humanity," Mo Gawdat, #Onebillionhappy (accessed December 10, 2018), https://www.onebillionhappy.org/happiness-library/mo-gawdats-moonshot-for-humanity-interview-part-i/.

37 Shawn Achor, "Positive Intelligence," *Harvard Business Review* 90, no. 1 (2012): 100–102; Sonja Lyubomirsky, Laura King, and Ed Diener, "The Benefits of Frequent Positive Affect: Does Happiness Lead to Success?," *Psychological Bulletin* 131, no. 6 (2005): 803.

38 Carol D. Ryff and Corey Lee M. Keyes, "The Structure of Psychological Well-Being Revisited," *Journal of Personality and Social Psychology* 69, no. 4 (1995): 719; Mitchell H. Gail, Jay H. Lubin, and Lawrence V. Rubinstein, "Likelihood Calculations for Matched Case-Control Studies and Survival Studies with Tied Death Times," *Biometrika* 68, no. 3 (1981): 703–7.

39 "The Science of Happiness at Work," Greater Good Science Center (accessed December 10, 2018), https://ggsc.berkeley.edu/what_we_do/online_courses_tools/the_science_of_happiness_at_work.

CHAPTER FIVE

1 Virginia A. Zakian, "Telomeres: The Beginnings and Ends of Eukaryotic Chromosomes," *Experimental Cell Research* 318, no. 12 (2012): 1456–60.

2 Elizabeth H. Blackburn and Joseph G. Gall, "A Tandemly Repeated Sequence at the Termini of the Extrachromosomal Ribosomal RNA Genes in Tetrahymena," *Journal of Molecular Biology* 120, no. 1 (1978): 33–53.

3 Ronald S. Petralia, Mark P. Mattson, and Pamela J. Yao, "Aging and Longevity in the Simplest Animals and the Quest for Immortality," *Ageing Research Reviews* 16 (2014): 66–82.

Notes

4   Richard M. Cawthon et al., "Association Between Telomere Length in Blood and Mortality in People Aged 60 Years or Older," *The Lancet* 361, no. 9355 (2003): 393–5.

5   Stephanie L. Bakaysa et al., "Telomere Length Predicts Survival Independent of Genetic Influences," *Aging Cell* 6, no. 6 (2007): 769–74.

6   Mario F. Fraga et al., "Epigenetic Differences Arise During the Lifetime of Monozygotic Twins," *Proceedings of the National Academy of Sciences* 102, no. 30 (2005): 10604–9.

7   Karl Lenhard Rudolph et al., "Longevity, Stress Response, and Cancer in Aging Telomerase-Deficient Mice," *Cell* 96, no. 5 (1999): 701–12; Erin M. Buckingham and Aloysius J. Klingelhutz, "The Role of Telomeres in the Ageing of Human Skin," *Experimental Dermatology* 20, no. 4 (2011): 297–302.

8   Dean Ornish et al., "Effect of Comprehensive Lifestyle Changes on Telomerase Activity and Telomere Length in Men With Biopsy-Proven Low-Risk Prostate Cancer: 5-Year Follow-Up of a Descriptive Pilot Study," *The Lancet Oncology* 14, no. 11 (2013): 1112–20; Dean Ornish et al., "Increased Telomerase Activity and Comprehensive Lifestyle Changes: A Pilot Study," *The Lancet Oncology* 9, no. 11 (2008): 1048–57.

9   Ed Diener and Micaela Y. Chan, "Happy People Live Longer: Subjective Well-Being Contributes to Health and Longevity," *Applied Psychology: Health and Well-Being* 3, no. 1 (2011): 1–43; Heather N. Rasmussen, Michael F. Scheier, and Joel B. Greenhouse, "Optimism and Physical Health: A Meta-Analytic Review," *Annals of Behavioral Medicine* 37, no. 3 (2009): 239–56.

10 Becca R. Levy et al., "Longevity Increased by Positive Self-Perceptions of Aging," *Journal of Personality and Social Psychology* 83, no. 2 (2002): 261.

11 Richard M. Ryan and Edward L. Deci, "On Happiness and Human Potentials: A Review of Research on Hedonic and Eudaimonic Well-Being," *Annual Review of Psychology* 52, no. 1 (2001): 141–66; Carol D. Ryff, Burton H. Singer, and Gayle Dienberg Love, "Positive Health: Connecting Well-Being with Biology," *Philosophical Transactions of the Royal Society B: Biological Sciences* 359, no. 1449 (2004): 1383.

12 Randy Cohen, Chirag Bavishi, and Alan Rozanski, "Purpose in Life and Its Relationship to All-Cause Mortality and Cardiovascular Events: A Meta-Analysis," *Psychosomatic Medicine* 78, no. 2 (2016): 122–33.

13 Megumi Koizumi et al., "Effect of Having a Sense of Purpose in Life on the Risk of Death from Cardiovascular Diseases," *Journal of Epidemiology* 18, no. 5 (2008): 191–96; Adam Kaplin and Laura Anzaldi, "New Movement in Neuroscience: A Purpose-Driven Life," *Cerebrum* 2015, no. 7 (May–June 2015).

14 Patricia A. Boyle et al., "Effect of a Purpose in Life on Risk of Incident Alzheimer Disease and Mild Cognitive Impairment in Community-Dwelling Older Persons," *Archives of General Psychiatry* 67, no. 3 (2010): 304–10.

15 Patricia A. Boyle et al., "Effect of Purpose in Life on the Relation Between Alzheimer Disease Pathologic Changes on Cognitive Function in Advanced Age," *Archives of General Psychiatry* 69, no. 5 (2012): 499–504.

16 "Paul Erdős: Hungarian Mathematician," Encyclopedia Britannica (accessed December 10, 2018), https://www.britannica.com/biography/Paul-Erdos.

17 "Obituary: Paul Erdős," *The London Times* (September 25, 1996), https://web.cs.elte.hu/erdos/London-Times.html.

18 Catherine E. Ross and Chia-ling Wu, "The Links Between Education and Health," *American Sociological Review* (1995): 719–45.

Notes

19   Jeannine S. Schiller, Jacqueline W. Lucas, and Jennifer A. Peregoy, "Summary Health Statistics for US Adults: National Health Interview Survey, 2011," *Vital Health Statistics* 10, no. 256 (2012): 1–218.

20   Marion Devaux et al., "Exploring the Relationship Between Education and Obesity," *OECD Journal: Economic Studies* 2011, no. 1 (2011): 1–40.

21   Alan R. Dyer et al., "The Relationship of Education to Blood Pressure: Findings on 40,000 Employed Chicagoans," *Circulation* 54, no. 6 (1976): 987–92.

22   Nancy Adler et al., "Educational Attainment and Late Life Telomere Length in the Health, Aging and Body Composition Study," *Brain, Behavior, and Immunity* 27 (2013): 15–21.

23   Patrick M. Krueger et al., "Mortality Attributable to Low Levels of Education in the United States," *PLOS ONE* 10, no. 7 (2015): e0131809.

24   Esther M. Friedman and Robert D. Mare, "The Schooling of Offspring and the Survival of Parents," *Demography* 51, no. 4 (2014): 1271–93.

25   S. Jay Olshansky et al., "Differences in Life Expectancy Due to Race and Educational Differences Are Widening, and Many May Not Catch Up," *Health Affairs* 31, no. 8 (2012): 1803–13; "Education: It Matters More to Health than Ever Before," Center on Society and Health, Virginia Commonwealth University (accessed December 11, 2018), https://societyhealth.vcu.edu/work/the-projects/education-it-matters-more -to-health-than-ever-before.html.

26   National Center for Health Statistics US, "Health, United States, 2011: With Special Feature on Socioeconomic Status and Health" (2012).

27   Emily B. Zimmerman et al., "The Case for Considering Education and Health," *Urban Education* 53, no. 6 (2018): 744–73.

28   Steven H. Woolf et al., "Giving Everyone the Health of the Educated: An Examination of Whether Social Change Would Save More Lives Than Medical Advances," *American Journal of Public Health* 97, no. 4 (2007): 679–83.

29   Angeline S. Lillard et al., "Montessori Preschool Elevates and Equalizes Child Outcomes: A Longitudinal Study," *Frontiers in Psychology* 8 (2017): 1783.

30   Leslie Morrison Gutman and John Vorhaus, "The Impact of Pupil Behaviour and Well-Being on Educational Outcomes," Lifelong Learning Platform (LLLPlatform) Position Paper (March 2012).

31   "Project ENGAGES (Engaging New Generations at Georgia Tech through Engineering & Science)," Parker H. Petit Institute for Bioengineering and Bioscience, Georgia Tech (accessed December 11, 2018), www.projectengages.gatech.edu.

32   Amanda Green, "The Incredible Story Behind the Senior Freshman Meme," *Refinery29* (updated December 1, 2016), https://www.refinery29.com/2016/09 /123998/senior-freshman-meme-nola-ochs.

33   Eric Klinenberg, *Palaces for the People: How Social Infrastructure Can Help Fight Inequality, Polarization, and the Decline of Civic Life* (New York: Crown Publishing Group, 2018).

34   "National Resource Center," Osher Lifelong Learning Institute (accessed December 11, 2018), http://nrc.northwestern.edu/.

35   "Explore Experiences," Airbnb (accessed December 11, 2018), https://www.airbnb .com/s/experiences?refinement_paths%5B%5D=%2Fexperiences.

Notes

CHAPTER SIX

1   "Oldest Goldfish Has His Chips," *BBC News* (August 7, 1999), http://news.bbc.co.uk
    /2/hi/uk/414114.stm.

2   Andrew Rundle et al., "The Urban Built Environment and Obesity in New York
    City: A Multilevel Analysis," *American Journal of Health Promotion* 21, no. 4, suppl.
    (2007): 326–34.

3   Sandro Galea, "Health in New York and Chicago by Subway and L-Stops: A Pictorial
    Essay," BU School of Public Health (May 17, 2015), https://www.bu.edu/sph/2015
    /05/17/health-in-new-york-and-chicago-by-subway-and-l-stops-a-pictorial-essay/;
    Nicolas M. Oreskovic et al., "Obesity and the Built Environment Among Massachu-
    setts Children," *Clinical Pediatrics* 48, no. 9 (2009): 904–12.

4   Andrew Rundle et al., "Neighborhood Food Environment and Walkability Predict
    Obesity in New York City," *Environmental Health Perspectives* 117, no. 3 (2008): 442–47.

5   Alisha Coleman-Jensen et al., "Statistical Supplement to Household Food Security in
    the United States in 2017," *US Department of Agriculture Economic Research Service*
    (2018).

6   Sam Dolnick, "The Obesity-Hunger Paradox," *New York Times* (March 12, 2010),
    https://www.nytimes.com/2010/03/14/nyregion/14hunger.html.

7   Alan Shenkin, "The Key Role of Micronutrients," *Clinical Nutrition* 25, no. 1 (2006):
    1–13.

8   Luke K. Ursell et al., "Defining the Human Microbiome," *Nutrition Reviews* 70,
    suppl. 1 (2012): S38–S44; Francesca de Filippis et al., "High-Level Adherence to a
    Mediterranean Diet Beneficially Impacts the Gut Microbiota and Associated Metab-
    olome," *Gut* 65, no. 11 (2016): 1812–21.

9   Vanessa K. Ridaura et al., "Gut Microbiota from Twins Discordant for Obesity Mod-
    ulate Metabolism in Mice," *Science* 341, no. 6150 (2013): 1241214.

10 James Collins et al., "Dietary Trehalose Enhances Virulence of Epidemic *Clostridium
    Difficile*," *Nature* 553, no. 7688 (2018): 291.

11 Daniel McDonald et al., "American Gut: An Open Platform for Citizen Science
    Microbiome Research," *mSystems* 3, no. 3 (2018): e00031–18.

12 Michael Lipsky, "How to Bring Farmers Markets to the Urban Poor," *The Wash-
    ington Post* (September 20, 2013), https://www.washingtonpost.com/opinions
    /how-to-bring-farmers-markets-to-the-urban-poor/2013/09/20/23cbe10c-14ac
    -11e3-880b-7503237cc69d_story.html?utm_term=.52bc624b3007.

13 Jim Latham and Tina Moffat, "Determinants of Variation in Food Cost and Avail-
    ability in Two Socioeconomically Contrasting Neighbourhoods of Hamilton, On-
    tario, Canada," *Health & Place* 13, no. 1 (2007): 273–87; Kristian Larsen and Jason
    Gilliland, "A Farmers' Market in a Food Desert: Evaluating Impacts on the Price and
    Availability of Healthy Food," *Health & Place* 15, no. 4 (2009): 1158–62.

14 Haoluan Wang, Feng Qiu, and Brent Swallow, "Can Community Gardens and Farm-
    ers' Markets Relieve Food Desert Problems? A Study of Edmonton, Canada," *Applied
    Geography* 55 (2014): 127–37.

15 Gail A. Langellotto and Abha Gupta, "Gardening Increases Vegetable Consumption
    in School-Aged Children: A Meta-Analytical Synthesis," *HortTechnology* 22, no. 4
    (2012): 430–45.

16 "Healthy Seedlings," Healthy Bodies, Healthy Gardens Curriculum, DUG (accessed
    December 12, 2018), https://dug.org/healthy-seedlings/.

Notes

17 Paige Pfleger, "Healthy Eaters, Strong Minds: What School Gardens Teach Kids," NPR (August 10, 2015), https://www.npr.org/sections/thesalt/2015/08/10/426741473/healthy-eaters-strong-minds-what-school-gardens-teach-kids.

18 Eugenia C. Garvin, Carolyn C. Cannuscio, and Charles C. Branas, "Greening Vacant Lots to Reduce Violent Crime: A Randomised Controlled Trial," *Injury Prevention* 19, no. 3 (2013): 198–203; Charles C. Branas et al., "Citywide Cluster Randomized Trial to Restore Blighted Vacant Land and Its Effects on Violence, Crime, and Fear," *Proceedings of the National Academy of Sciences* 15, no. 12 (2018): 2946–51.

19 "Detroit Grocery Incubator Project," Fair Food Network (accessed December 12, 2018), https://fairfoodnetwork.org/projects/detroit-grocery-incubator-project/.

20 Roland Sturm and Deborah A. Cohen, "Suburban Sprawl and Physical and Mental Health," *Public Health* 118, no. 7 (2004): 488–96.

21 James F. Sallis et al., "Physical Activity in Relation to Urban Environments in 14 Cities Worldwide: A Cross-Sectional Study," *The Lancet* 387, no. 10034 (2016): 2207–17.

22 Michelle L. Bell, Devra L. Davis, and Tony Fletcher, "A Retrospective Assessment of Mortality from the London Smog Episode of 1952: The Role of Influenza and Pollution," *Environmental Health Perspectives* 112, no. 1 (2004): 6.

23 Francine Laden et al., "Reduction in Fine Particulate Air Pollution and Mortality: Extended Follow-Up of the Harvard Six Cities Study," *American Journal of Respiratory and Critical Care Medicine* 173, no. 6 (2006): 667–72.

24 Joshua S. Apte et al., "Ambient PM2.5 Reduces Global and Regional Life Expectancy," *Environmental Science & Technology Letters* 5, no. 9 (2018): 546–51; Kelly C. Bishop et al., *Hazed and Confused: The Effect of Air Pollution on Dementia*, no. w24970. National Bureau of Economic Research (2018).

25 Qian Di et al., "Association of Short-Term Exposure to Air Pollution With Mortality in Older Adults," *JAMA* 318, no. 24 (2017): 2446–56.

26 Jaime E. Hart et al., "Roadway Proximity and Risk of Sudden Cardiac Death in Women," *Circulation* (2014), https://www.ahajournals.org/doi/full/10.1161/CIRCULATIONAHA.114.011489].

27 Monica S. Hammer, Tracy K. Swinburn, and Richard L. Neitzel, "Environmental Noise Pollution in the United States: Developing an Effective Public Health Response," *Environmental Health Perspectives* 122, no. 2 (2013): 115–19.

28 Mathew P. White et al., "Would You Be Happier Living in a Greener Urban Area? A Fixed-Effects Analysis of Panel Data," *Psychological Science* 24, no. 6 (2013): 920–28.

29 Ralf Hansmann, Stella-Maria Hug, and Klaus Seeland, "Restoration and Stress Relief Through Physical Activities in Forests and Parks," *Urban Forestry & Urban Greening* 6, no. 4 (2007): 213–25.

30 Roland Sturm and Deborah Cohen, "Proximity to Urban Parks and Mental Health," *The Journal of Mental Health Policy and Economics* 17, no. 1 (2014): 19; Marc G. Berman et al., "Interacting with Nature Improves Cognition and Affect for Individuals With Depression," *Journal of Affective Disorders* 140, no. 3 (2012): 300–5.

31 Mark S. Taylor et al., "Research Note: Urban Street Tree Density and Antidepressant Prescription Rates—A Cross-Sectional Study in London, UK," *Landscape and Urban Planning* 136 (2015): 174–79.

32 Mathew P. White et al., "Would You Be Happier Living in a Greener Urban Area?"

33 Qing Li et al., "A Forest Bathing Trip Increases Human Natural Killer Activity and Expression of Anti-Cancer Proteins in Female Subjects," *Journal of Biological Regulators Homeostatic Agents* 22, no. 1 (2008): 45–55.

34 Qing Li, "Effect of Forest Bathing Trips on Human Immune Function," *Environmental Health and Preventive Medicine* 15, no. 1 (2010): 9.

35 Roger S. Ulrich, "View Through a Window May Influence Recovery From Surgery," *Science* 224, no. 4647 (1984): 420–21.

36 Nancy M. Wells and Gary W. Evans, "Nearby Nature: A Buffer of Life Stress Among Rural Children," *Environment and Behavior* 35, no. 3 (2003): 311–30; K. Dijkstra, Marcel E. Pieterse, and A. Pruyn, "Stress-Reducing Effects of Indoor Plants in the Built Healthcare Environment: The Mediating Role of Perceived Attractiveness," *Preventive Medicine* 47, no. 3 (2008): 279–83.

37 "Brownsville," Crime and Safety Report, DNAinfo (accessed December 13, 2018), https://www.dnainfo.com/crime-safety-report/brooklyn/brownsville/.

38 "Home Owners' Loan Corporation," Dictionary of American History, Encyclopedia .com (January 12, 2019), https://www.encyclopedia.com/history/dictionaries-thesauruses-pictures-and-press-releases/home-owners-loan-corporation.

39 Robert K. Nelson et al., "Mapping Inequality," *American Panorama*, ed. Robert K. Nelson and Edward L. Ayers (accessed December 13, 2018), https://dsl.richmond .edu/panorama/redlining/#loc=4/36.71/-96.93&opacity=0.8.

40 "Brownsville, Brooklyn, NY," *Redlining Virginia* (accessed December 10, 2018), http://www.redliningvirginia.org/exhibits/show/the-national-story/item/1.

41 "Country Comparison: Infant Mortality Rate," *The World Factbook*, Central Intelligence Agency, https://www.cia.gov/library/publications/the-world-factbook /rankorder/2091rank.html.

42 Wilhelmine Miller, Patti Simon, and Saqi Maleque, "Beyond Health Care: New Directions to a Healthier America," Robert Wood Johnson Foundation Commission to Build a Healthier America (April 2009).

43 J. L. Christopher et al., "Eight Americas: Investigating Mortality Disparities Across Races, Counties, and Race-Counties in the United States," *PLOS Medicine* 3, no. 9 (2006): e260.

44 "Mapping Life Expectancy: Washington, D.C." Center on Society and Health, Virginia Commonwealth University in partnership with RWJF Commission to Build a Healthier America (accessed December 11, 2018), https://societyhealth.vcu.edu /work/the-projects/mapswashingtondc.html.

45 Michael Marmot, "The Status Syndrome: How Social Standing Affects Our Health and Longevity" (London: Bloomsbury, 2004).

46 Katherine P. Theall et al., "Neighborhood Disorder and Telomeres: Connecting Children's Exposure to Community Level Stress and Cellular Response," *Social Science & Medicine* 85 (2013): 50–58.

47 Latetia V. Moore and Ana V. Diez Roux, "Associations of Neighborhood Characteristics with the Location and Type of Food Stores," *American Journal of Public Health* 96, no. 2 (2006): 325–31.

48 Michael Marmot, "The Status Syndrome" (2004).

49 Mindy Thompson Fullilove and Rodrick Wallace, "Serial Forced Displacement in American Cities, 1916–2010," *Journal of Urban Health* 88, no. 3 (2011): 381–89.

50 Greenleaf Housing Community Co-developer RFQ, District of Columbia Housing Authority (issued December 18, 2018), http://www.dchousing.org/docs/2017 121810073284810.pdf.

51 Mindy Fullilove (public psychiatrist, author, and professor of Urban Policy and Health at The New School), in discussion with the author (May 2016).

Notes

52 Patrick Sharkey, Gerard Torrats-Espinosa, and Delaram Takyar, "Community and the Crime Decline: The Causal Effect of Local Nonprofits on Violent Crime," *American Sociological Review* 82, no. 6 (2017): 1214–40.

53 Charles C. Branas et al., "Urban Blight Remediation as a Cost-Beneficial Solution to Firearm Violence," *American Journal of Public Health* 106, no. 12 (2016): 2158–64.

54 "Evidence of Success," Pennsylvania Horticultural Society (accessed December 13, 2018), https://phsonline.org/programs/landcare-program/evidence-of-success/.

55 Yasmeen Khan, "Brownsville: No Label Necessary," WNYC (January 29, 2018), https://www.wnyc.org/story/brownsville-no-label-necessary/.

56 Anand Giridharadas, "Exploring New York, Unplugged and on Foot," *New York Times* (January 24, 2013), https://www.nytimes.com/2013/01/25/nyregion/exploring-red-hook-brooklyn-unplugged-and-with-friends.html.

57 "Organizing Your Own," #IamHere Days (accessed December 13, 2018), http://iamheredays.tumblr.com.

58 Sandro Galea et al., "Estimated Deaths Attributable to Social Factors in the United States," *American Journal of Public Health* 101, no. 8 (2011): 1456–65.

59 "Starting a Farmers' Market," University of Florida (April 2014), http://sfyl.ifas.ufl.edu/agriculture/starting-a-farmers-market/.

CHAPTER SEVEN

1 Helen Shen, "Mind the Gender Gap," *Nature* 495, no. 7439 (2013): 22.

2 Corinne A. Moss-Racusin et al., "Science Faculty's Subtle Gender Biases Favor Male Students," *Proceedings of the National Academy of Sciences* 109, no. 41 (2012): 16474–79.

3 Scott Decker et al., "Criminal Stigma, Race, Gender, and Employment: An Expanded Assessment of the Consequences of Imprisonment for Employment," Department of Justice (2014), https://www.ncjrs.gov/pdffiles1/nij/grants/244756.pdf.

4 Marianne Bertrand and Sendhil Mullainathan, "Are Emily and Greg More Employable Than Lakisha and Jamal? A Field Experiment on Labor Market Discrimination," *American Economic Review* 94, no. 4 (2004): 991–1013.

5 Daniel Widner and Stephen Chicoine, "It's All in the Name: Employment Discrimination Against Arab Americans 1," In *Sociological Forum*, vol. 26, no. 4 (2011): 806–23 (Oxford, UK: Blackwell Publishing Ltd., 2011).

6 Marianne Bertrand and Sendhil Mullainathan, "Are Emily and Greg More Employable Than Lakisha and Jamal? A Field Experiment on Labor Market Discrimination," *American Economic Review* 94, no. 4 (2004): 991–1013.

7 "Income and Poverty in the United States: 2016," Report Number P60-259, US Census Bureau (updated September 12, 2017), https://www.census.gov/library/publications/2017/demo/p60-259.html.

8 Kim Parker and Cary Funk, "Gender Discrimination Comes in Many Forms for Today's Working Women," Pew Research Center (December 14, 2017), http://www.pewresearch.org/fact-tank/2017/12/14/gender-discrimination-comes-in-many-forms-for-todays-working-women/.

9 "Fact Sheet: Black Women and the Wage Gap," National Partnership for Women & Families (April 2018), http://www.nationalpartnership.org/our-work/resources/workplace/fair-pay/african-american-women-wage-gap.pdf.

Notes

10 "The Gender Wage Gap in NYC," New York City Comptroller (updated August 3, 2018), https://comptroller.nyc.gov/reports/gender-wage-gap/inside-the-gender-wage -gap/inside-the-gender-wage-gap-part-i-earnings-of-black-women-in-new-york-city/.

11 Andrea Mandell, "Exclusive: Wahlberg got $1.5M for 'All the Money' Reshoot, Williams Paid Less than $1,000," USA Today (January 9, 2018), https://www.usa today.com/story/life/people/2018/01/09/exclusive-wahlberg-paid-1-5-m-all -money-reshoot-williams-got-less-than-1-000/1018351001/.

12 Julie Anderson, Jessica Milli, and Melanie Kruvelis, "Projected Year the Wage Gap Will Close by State," Institute for Women's Policy Research (March 22, 2017), https:// iwpr.org/publications/projected-year-wage-gap-will-close-state/.

13 "Wyoming Facts and Symbols," State of Wyoming (accessed January 20, 2019), http://www.wyo.gov/about-wyoming/wyoming-facts-and-symbols; "The Global Gender Gap Report 2018," World Economic Forum (accessed January 20, 2019), http://reports.weforum.org/global-gender-gap-report-2018/.

14 Ronald C. Kessler et al., "Prevalence, Severity, and Comorbidity of 12-Month DSM-IV Disorders in the National Comorbidity Survey Replication," Archives of General Psychiatry 62, no. 6 (2005): 617–27; Oriana Vesga-López et al., "Gender Differences in Generalized Anxiety Disorder: Results from the National Epidemiologic Survey on Alcohol and Related Conditions (NESARC)," Journal of Clinical Psychiatry 69, no. 10 (2008): 1606.

15 Jonathan Platt et al., "Unequal Depression for Equal Work? How the Wage Gap Explains Gendered Disparities in Mood Disorders," Social Science & Medicine 149 (2016): 1–8.

16 Richard G. Wilkinson and Kate E. Pickett, "Income Inequality and Population Health: A Review and Explanation of the Evidence," Social Science & Medicine 62, no. 7 (2006): 1768–84.

17 Haidong Wang et al., "Age-Specific and Sex-Specific Mortality in 187 Countries, 1970–2010: A Systematic Analysis for the Global Burden of Disease Study 2010," The Lancet 380, no. 9859 (2012): 2071–94.

18 Shane A. Kavanagh, Julia M. Shelley, and Christopher Stevenson, "Does Gender Inequity Increase Men's Mortality Risk in the United States? A Multilevel Analysis of Data from the National Longitudinal Mortality Study," SSM-Population Health 3 (2017): 358–65.

19 Uri Leviatan and Jiska Cohen, "Gender Differences in Life Expectancy Among Kibbutz Members," Social Science & Medicine 21, no. 5 (1985): 545–51.

20 Arline T. Geronimus, "The Weathering Hypothesis and the Health of African-American Women and Infants: Evidence and Speculations," Ethnicity & Disease 2, no. 3 (1992): 207–21.

21 Ichiro Kawachi et al., "Women's Status and the Health of Women and Men: A View from the States," Social Science & Medicine 48, no. 1 (1999): 21–32; Øystein Gullvåg Holter, "What's in It for Men? Old Question, New Data," Men and Masculinities 17, no. 5 (2014): 515–48.

22 Zinzi D. Bailey et al., "Structural Racism and Health Inequities in the USA: Evidence and Interventions," The Lancet 389, no. 10077 (2017): 1453–63.

23 Anthony G. Greenwald and Linda Hamilton Krieger, "Implicit Bias: Scientific Foundations," California Law Review 94, no. 4 (2006): 945–67.

24 Ronald M. Epstein and Edward M. Hundert, "Defining and Assessing Professional Competence," JAMA 287, no. 2 (2002): 226–35.

25 Edward M. Hundert, Darleen Douglas-Steele, and Janet Bickel, "Context in Medical Education: The Informal Ethics Curriculum," *Medical Education* 30, no. 5 (1996): 353–64.

26 Rachel L. Johnson et al., "Patient Race/Ethnicity and Quality of Patient–Physician Communication During Medical Visits," *American Journal of Public Health* 94, no. 12 (2004): 2084–90.

27 Kevin A. Schulman et al., "The Effect of Race and Sex on Physicians' Recommendations for Cardiac Catheterization," *New England Journal of Medicine* 340, no. 8 (1999): 618–26.

28 Janice A. Sabin, Rachel G. Riskind, and Brian A. Nosek, "Health-Care Providers' Implicit and Explicit Attitudes Toward Lesbian Women and Gay Men," *American Journal of Public Health* 105, no. 9 (2015): 1831–41.

29 Christopher T. Richards, LaVera M. Crawley, and David Magnus, "Use of Neurodevelopmental Delay in Pediatric Solid Organ Transplant Listing Decisions: Inconsistencies in Standards Across Major Pediatric Transplant Centers," *Pediatric Transplantation* 13, no. 7 (2009): 843–50; Jackie Fortier, "People With Developmental Disabilities May Face Organ Transplant Bias," State Impact Oklahoma Report, NPR (March 15, 2018), https://stateimpact.npr.org/oklahoma/2018/03/15/people-with-developmental-disabilities-may-face-organ-transplant-bias/.

30 Sean M. Phelan et al., "Impact of Weight Bias and Stigma on Quality of Care and Outcomes for Patients with Obesity," *Obesity Reviews* 16, no. 4 (2015): 319–26.

31 Stephanie Knaak, Ed Mantler, and Andrew Szeto, "Mental Illness–Related Stigma in Healthcare: Barriers to Access and Care and Evidence-Based Solutions," *Healthcare Management Forum* 30, no. 2 (2017): 111–16.

32 Ribhi Hazin, "The Protest Psychosis: How Schizophrenia Became a Black Disease," *Journal of the National Medical Association* 103, no. 4 (2011): 375; Robert C. Schwartz and David M. Blankenship, "Racial Disparities in Psychotic Disorder Diagnosis: A Review of Empirical Literature," *World Journal of Psychiatry* 4, no. 4 (2014): 133.

33 Adil H. Haider et al., "Race and Insurance Status as Risk Factors for Trauma Mortality," *Archives of Surgery* 143, no. 10 (2008): 945–49.

34 Elissa Ely, "Dr. Understood Racism on Multiple Fronts," The Remembrance Project, WBUR (accessed December 13, 2018), http://www.wbur.org/remembrance-project/2017/02/08/dr-chester-pierce.

35 "Dr. Derald Wing Sue," American Psychological Association (accessed December 13, 2018), http://www.apa.org/pi/oema/resources/ethnicity-health/psychologists/derald-wing-sue.aspx.

36 Derald Wing Sue et al., "Racial Microaggressions in Everyday Life: Implications for Clinical Practice," *American Psychologist* 62, no. 4 (2007): 271.

37 "Microaggressions: Power, Privilege, and Everyday Life." The Microaggressions Project (accessed December 13, 2018), http://www.microaggressions.com/.

38 Christina B. Chin et al., "Tokens on the Small Screen: Asian Americans and Pacific Islanders in Prime Time and Streaming Television" (accessed December 13, 2018), http://www.aapisontv.com/uploads/3/8/1/3/38136681/aapisontv.2017.pdf.

39 "Low Birthweight," March of Dimes (accessed December 13, 2018), https://www.marchofdimes.org/baby/low-birthweight.aspx.

40 Diane S. Lauderdale, "Birth Outcomes for Arabic-Named Women in California Before and After September 11," *Demography* 43, no. 1 (2006): 185–201.

41 "Brown at 60," NAACP, Legal Defense and Education Fund (accessed August 15, 2017), http://www.naacpldf.org/brown-at-60-the-doll-test.

Notes

42 Kenneth B. Clark and Mamie Phipps Clark, "C250 Celebrates Columbians Ahead of Their Time," Columbia University (accessed January 11, 2019), http://c250.colum bia.edu/c250_celebrates/remarkable_columbians/kenneth_mamie_clark.html.

43 Abraham L. Davis, *The United States Supreme Court and the Uses of Social Science Data* (New York: Ardent Media, 1973), 53.

44 Stephen J. Dubner, "Why Does a Caucasian Dollhouse Cost Nearly 70% More Than an African-American Dollhouse?" (December 2, 2011), http://freakonomics .com/2011/12/02/why-does-a-caucasian-dollhouse-cost-nearly-70-more-than-an -african-american-dollhouse/.

45 Margaret Beale Spencer, "Study: White and Black Children Biased Toward Lighter Skin," CNN, AC360 (May 14, 2010), http://www.cnn.com/2010/US/05/13/doll.study /index.html.

46 Anthony G. Greenwald et al., "Understanding and Using the Implicit Association Test: III. Meta-Analysis of Predictive Validity." *Journal of Personality and Social Psychology* 97, no. 1 (2009): 17.

47 Earle C. Chambers et al., "The Relationship of Internalized Racism to Body Fat Distribution and Insulin Resistance Among African Adolescent Youth," *Journal of the National Medical Association* 96, no. 12 (2004): 1594.

48 Jerome Taylor and Beryl Jackson, "Factors Affecting Alcohol Consumption in Black Women Part II," *International Journal of the Addictions* 25, no. 12 (1990): 1415–27.

49 David H. Chae et al., "Discrimination, Racial Bias, and Telomere Length in African-American Men," *American Journal of Preventive Medicine* 46, no. 2 (2014): 103–11.

50 Alexander R. Green et al., "Implicit Bias Among Physicians and Its Prediction of Thrombolysis Decisions for Black and White Patients," *Journal of General Internal Medicine* 22, no. 9 (2007): 1231–38.

51 Claude M. Steele, "Thin Ice: Stereotype Threat and Black College Students," *The Atlantic* (August 1999), https://www.theatlantic.com/magazine/archive/1999/08 /thin-ice-stereotype-threat-and-black-college-students/304663/.

52 Claude M. Steele and Joshua Aronson, "Stereotype Threat and the Intellectual Test Performance of African Americans," *Journal of Personality and Social Psychology* 69, no. 5 (1995): 797.

53 Joshua Aronson et al., "Unhealthy Interactions: The Role of Stereotype Threat in Health Disparities," *American Journal of Public Health* 103, no. 1 (2013): 50–56.

54 Steven Spencer, Claude M. Steele, and Diane M. Quinn, "Stereotype Threat and Women's Math Performance," *Journal of Experimental Social Psychology* 35, no. 1 (1999): 4–28; Toni Schmader and Michael Johns, "Converging Evidence that Stereotype Threat Reduces Working Memory Capacity," *Journal of Personality and Social Psychology* 85, no. 3 (2003): 440; Brian Armenta, "Stereotype Boost and Stereotype Threat Effects: The Moderating Role of Ethnic Identification," *Cultural Diversity and Ethnic Minority Psychology* 16, no. 1 (2010): 94.

55 Jean-Claude Croizet et al., "Stereotype Threat Undermines Intellectual Performance by Triggering a Disruptive Mental Load," *Personality and Social Psychology Bulletin* 30, no. 6 (2004): 721–31.

56 Jim Blascovich et al., "African Americans and High Blood Pressure: The Role of Stereotype Threat," *Psychological Science* 12, no. 3 (2001): 225–9.

57 Tené T. Lewis et al., "Self-Reported Experiences of Everyday Discrimination Are Associated With Elevated C-Reactive Protein Levels in Older African-American Adults," *Brain, Behavior, and Immunity* 24, no. 3 (2010): 438–43.

58   Kenneth C. Schoendorf et al., "Mortality Among Infants of Black as Compared With White College-Educated Parents," *New England Journal of Medicine* 326, no. 23 (1992): 1522–26; Corinne A. Riddell, Sam Harper, and Jay S. Kaufman, "Trends in Differences in US Mortality Rates Between Black and White Infants," *JAMA Pediatrics* 171, no. 9 (2017): 911–13.

59   Richard V. Reeves and Davna Bowen Matthew, "Social Mobility Memos: 6 Charts Showing Race Gaps Within the American Middle Class," Brookings Institution (October 21, 2016), https://www.brookings.edu/blog/social-mobility-memos/2016/10/21/6-charts-showing-race-gaps-within-the-american-middle-class/.

60   Larry Adelman, *Race: The Power of an Illusion*, California Newsreel: USA (2003), http://www.pbs.org/race/000_General/000_00-Home.htm.

61   Francis S. Collins and Monique K. Mansoura, "The Human Genome Project: Revealing the Shared Inheritance of All Humankind," *Cancer: Interdisciplinary International Journal of the American Cancer Society* 91, no. S1 (2001): 221–5.

62   "DNA Discussion Project," West Chester University (accessed December 15, 2018), https://www.wcupa.edu/dnaDiscussion/about.aspx.

63   "Division of Tribal Government Services," US Department of the Interior, Indian Affairs (accessed January 20, 2019), https://www.bia.gov/bia/ois/tgs/genealogy.

64   Dorothy Roberts, "The Problem With Race-Based Medicine," filmed November 2015 at TEDMed.https://www.ted.com/talks/dorothy_roberts_the_problem_with_race_based_medicine.

65   Cynthia García Coll and Amy Kerivan Marks, eds., *The Immigrant Paradox in Children and Adolescents: Is Becoming American a Developmental Risk?* (Washington, DC: American Psychological Association, 2012); Leslie O. Schulz et al., "Effects of Traditional and Western Environments on Prevalence of Type 2 Diabetes in Pima Indians in Mexico and the US," *Diabetes Care* 29, no. 8 (2006): 1866–71.

66   Edna A. Viruell-Fuentes, Patricia Y. Miranda, and Sawsan Abdulrahim, "More Than Culture: Structural Racism, Intersectionality Theory, and Immigrant Health," *Social Science & Medicine* 75, no. 12 (2012): 2099–106.

67   David Squires and Chloe Anderson, "US Health Care from a Global Perspective: Spending, Use of Services, Prices, and Health in 13 Countries," *The Commonwealth Fund* 15, no. 3 (2015): 1–16; Mauricio Avendano and Ichiro Kawachi, "Why Do Americans Have Shorter Life Expectancy and Worse Health Than Do People in Other High-Income Countries?" *Annual Review of Public Health* 35 (2014): 307–25.

68   Renato D. Alarcón et al., "Hispanic Immigrants in the USA: Social and Mental Health Perspectives," *The Lancet Psychiatry* 3, no. 9 (2016): 860–70.

69   Giorgia Silani et al., "Right Supramarginal Gyrus Is Crucial to Overcome Emotional Egocentricity Bias in Social Judgments," *Journal of Neuroscience* 33, no. 39 (2013): 15466–76.

70   James F. Cavanagh et al., "Frontal Theta Overrides Pavlovian Learning Biases," *Journal of Neuroscience* 33, no. 19 (2013): 8541–48.

71   "Meditation on Loving Kindness," Jack Kornfield (accessed January 23, 2019), https://jackkornfield.com/meditation-on-lovingkindness/.

72   Rupert Brown and Miles Hewstone, "An Integrative Theory of Intergroup Contact," *Advances in Experimental Social Psychology* 37, no. 37 (2005): 255–343; Thomas F. Pettigrew and Linda R. Tropp, "A Meta-Analytic Test of Intergroup Contact Theory," *Journal of Personality and Social Psychology* 90, no. 5 (2006): 751.

73   Patricia G. Devine et al., "Long-Term Reduction in Implicit Race Bias: A Prejudice

Habit-Breaking Intervention," *Journal of Experimental Social Psychology* 48, no. 6 (2012): 1267–78.

74 Molly Carnes et al., "Effect of an Intervention to Break the Gender Bias Habit for Faculty at One Institution: A Cluster Randomized, Controlled Trial," *Academic Medicine: Journal of the Association of American Medical Colleges* 90, no. 2 (2015): 221; Patricia G. Devine et al., "A Gender Bias Habit-Breaking Intervention Led to Increased Hiring of Female Faculty in STEMM Departments," *Journal of Experimental Social Psychology* 73 (2017): 211–15.

75 Patricia G. Devine et al., "Long-Term Reduction in Implicit Race Bias."

76 Tim Halloran, "How Johnson & Johnson Is Adding 90,000 More Women to Their Hiring Pipeline" (accessed December 18, 2018), https://textio.ai/johnson-and -johnson-textio-video-d95c1480c601.

77 Patricia G. Devine, "Empowering People to Break the Prejudice Habit" (May 6, 2018), https://madison.com/wsj/discovery/empowering-people-to-break-the -prejudice-habit/article_7afd069e-97a7-5011-844e-56f3fc25c3d0.html; Jessica Nordell, "Is This How Discrimination Ends?" *The Atlantic* (May 7, 2017), https://www .theatlantic.com/science/archive/2017/05/unconscious-bias-training/525405/.

CHAPTER EIGHT

1 Cezara Anton, "How Did the Second World War Affect the British Society," *Historia* (accessed December 18, 2018), https://www.historia.ro/sectiune/general/articol /how-did-the-second-world-war-affect-the-british-society.

2 Richard Doll and A. Bradford Hill, "Smoking and Carcinoma of the Lung," *BMJ* 2, no. 4682 (1950): 739.

3 Michael J. Thun, "When Truth Is Unwelcome: The First Reports on Smoking and Lung Cancer," *Bulletin of the World Health Organization* 83 (2005): 144–45.

4 Ernst L. Wynder, MD, "Morbidity and Mortality Weekly Report, Centers for Disease Control (November 5, 1999), https://www.cdc.gov/mmwr/preview/mmwrhtml /mm4843bx.htm.

5 Caroline Richmond, "Sir Richard Doll," *The BMJ* (accessed December 18, 2018), https://www.bmj.com/content/suppl/2005/07/28/331.7511.295.DC1.

6 Ernst L. Wynder and Evarts A. Graham, "Tobacco Smoking as a Possible Etiologic Factor in Bronchogenic Carcinoma," *JAMA* 143 (1950): 329–36.

7 Doll and Hill, "Smoking and Carcinoma of the Lung."

8 CDC, "Ernst L. Wynder, MD."

9 Richmond, "Sir Richard Doll."

10 CDC, "Ernst L. Wynder, MD."

11 Jane Ellen Stevens, "The Adverse Childhood Experiences Study—The Largest, Most Important Public Health Study You Never Heard Of—Began in an Obesity Clinic," *ACES Too High News* 3 (2012).

12 Vincent Felitti, interview in "Resilience: The Biology of Stress and the Science of Hope," directed by James Redford, KPJR Films (2016), https://kpjrfilms.co/resilience/.

13 Bessel A. Van der Kolk, "The Body Keeps the Score: Memory and the Evolving Psychobiology of Posttraumatic Stress," *Harvard Review of Psychiatry* 1, no. 5 (1994): 253–65.

14 Vincent J. Felitti et al., "Relationship of Childhood Abuse and Household Dysfunction

to Many of the Leading Causes of Death in Adults: The Adverse Childhood Experiences (ACE) Study," *American Journal of Preventive Medicine* 14, no. 4 (1998): 245–58.

15 Robert F. Anda et al., "Adverse Childhood Experiences and Chronic Obstructive Pulmonary Disease in Adults," *American Journal of Preventive Medicine* 34, no. 5 (2008): 396–403; Maxia Dong et al., "Insights into Causal Pathways for Ischemic Heart Disease: Adverse Childhood Experiences Study," *Circulation* 110, no. 13 (2004): 1761–66.

16 Vincent Felitti et al., "Relationship of Childhood Abuse and Household Dysfunction to Many of the Leading Causes of Death in Adults."

17 David W. Brown et al., "Adverse Childhood Experiences Are Associated With the Risk of Lung Cancer: A Prospective Cohort Study," *BMC Public Health* 10, no. 1 (2010): 20.

18 "Toxic Stress," Center on the Developing Child, Harvard University (accessed December 18, 2018), https://developingchild.harvard.edu/science/key-concepts/toxic-stress/.

19 Shanta R. Dube et al., "Childhood Abuse, Household Dysfunction, and the Risk of Attempted Suicide Throughout the Life Span: Findings From the Adverse Childhood Experiences Study," *JAMA* 286, no. 24 (2001): 3089–96.

20 Sally A. Moore, Lori A. Zoellner, and Niklas Mollenholt, "Are Expressive Suppression and Cognitive Reappraisal Associated With Stress-Related Symptoms?," *Behaviour Research and Therapy* 46, no. 9 (2008): 993–1000.

21 Allison S. Troy et al., "Seeing the Silver Lining: Cognitive Reappraisal Ability Moderates the Relationship Between Stress and Depressive Symptoms," *Emotion* 10, no. 6 (2010): 783.

22 "DBT: An Evidence-Based Treatment," Behavioral Tech: A Linehan Institute Training Company (accessed December 26, 2018), https://behavioraltech.org/research/; Benedict Carey, "Expert on Mental Illness Reveals Her Own Fight," *New York Times* (June 23, 2011).

23 "The Wound Is the Place Where the Light Enters" (accessed December 26, 2018), https://mettahu.wordpress.com/2014/02/13/the-wound-is-the-place-where-the-light-enters/.

24 "What Is PTG?" Posttraumatic Growth Research Group, UNC Charlotte (accessed December 18, 2018), https://ptgi.uncc.edu/what-is-ptg/.

25 Shirley A. Murphy, L. Clark Johnson, and Janet Lohan, "Finding Meaning in a Child's Violent Death: A Five-Year Prospective Analysis of Parents' Personal Narratives and Empirical Data," *Death Studies* 27, no. 5 (2003): 381–404.

26 James W. Pennebaker, Janice K. Kiecolt-Glaser, and Ronald Glaser, "Disclosure of Traumas and Immune Function: Health Implications for Psychotherapy," *Journal of Consulting and Clinical Psychology* 56, no. 2 (1988): 239.

27 James W. Pennebaker and Janel D. Seagal, "Forming a Story: The Health Benefits of Narrative," *Journal of Clinical Psychology* 55, no. 10 (1999): 1243–54.

28 Meredith Edgar-Bailey and Victoria E. Kress, "Resolving Child and Adolescent Traumatic Grief: Creative Techniques and Interventions," *Journal of Creativity in Mental Health* 5, no. 2 (2010): 158–76; Heather L. Stuckey and Jeremy Nobel, "The Connection Between Art, Healing, and Public Health: A Review of Current Literature," *American Journal of Public Health* 100, no. 2 (2010): 254–63.

29 Beulah Amsterdam, "Mirror Self-Image Reactions Before Age Two," *Developmental Psychobiology* 5, no. 4 (1972): 297–305.

30 Lamei Wang, Liqi Zhu, and Zhenlin Wang, "The Role of Theory of Mind and Inhibitory Control in Children's Social Functioning: Practical Joke and Keeping a Secret," Conference Paper (2014), https://www.researchgate.net/publication

/276028012_The_role_of_theory_of_mind_and_inhibitory_control_in_children's
_social_functioning_Practical_joke_and_keeping_a_secret.

31 Paul Bloom, "The Moral Life of Babies," *New York Times Magazine* 3 (2010).

32 Olga M. Klimecki et al., "Differential Pattern of Functional Brain Plasticity After Compassion and Empathy Training," *Social Cognitive and Affective Neuroscience* 9, no. 6 (2013): 873–79.

33 James M. Kilner and Roger N. Lemon, "What We Know Currently About Mirror Neurons," *Current Biology* 23, no. 23 (2013): r1057–r1062.

34 Bahar Tunçgenç and Emma Cohen, "Interpersonal Movement Synchrony Facilitates Pro-Social Behavior in Children's Peer-Play," *Developmental Science* 21, no. 1 (2018): e12505.

35 Sourya Acharya and Samarth Shukla, "Mirror Neurons: Enigma of the Metaphysical Modular Brain," *Journal of Natural Science, Biology, and Medicine* 3, no. 2 (2012): 118.

36 Helen Wilkinson et al., "Examining the Relationship Between Burnout and Empathy in Healthcare Professionals: A Systematic Review," *Burnout Research* 6 (2017): 18–29.

37 Jeffrey M. Lohr at al., "The Psychology of Anger Venting and Empirically Supported Alternatives That Do No Harm," *Scientific Review of Mental Health Practice* 5, no. 1 (2007).

38 Ryan W. Carpenter and Timothy J. Trull, "Components of Emotion Dysregulation in Borderline Personality Disorder: A Review," *Current Psychiatry Reports* 15, no. 1 (2013): 335.

39 Benedetta Vai et al., "Corticolimbic Connectivity Mediates the Relationship Between Adverse Childhood Experiences and Symptom Severity in Borderline Personality Disorder," *Neuropsychobiology* 76, no. 2 (2017): 105–15.

40 Mary C. Zanarini et al., "Prediction of the 10-Year Course of Borderline Personality Disorder," *American Journal of Psychiatry* 163, no. 5 (2006): 827–32.

41 Lucas Fortaleza de Aquino Ferreira et al., "Borderline Personality Disorder and Sexual Abuse: A Systematic Review," *Psychiatry Research* 262 (2018): 70–77.

42 Cameron Hancock, "The Stigma Associated With Borderline Personality Disorder," NAMI (June 28, 2017), https://www.nami.org/Blogs/NAMI-Blog/June-2017 /The-Stigma-Associated-with-Borderline-Personality.

43 Center for Substance Abuse Treatment, "Trauma-Informed Care in Behavioral Health Services" (2014), [Appendix C], https://www.ncbi.nlm.nih.gov/pubmed /24901203.

44 "Trauma Training for Criminal Justice Professionals," SAMHSA (updated August 19, 2015), https://www.samhsa.gov/gains-center/trauma-training-criminal-justice -professionals.

45 V. J. Felitti et al., "The Adverse Childhood Experiences (ACE) Study."

46 "Adverse Childhood Experience (ACE) Questionnaire: Finding Your ACE Score" (accessed December 30, 2018), https://www.ncjfcj.org/sites/default/files/Finding %20Your%20ACE%20Score.pdf.

CHAPTER NINE

1 Mark L. Graber, Robert M. Wachter, and Christine K. Cassel, "Bringing Diagnosis Into the Quality and Safety Equations," *JAMA* 308, no. 12 (2012): 1211–12; Bradford Winters et al., "Diagnostic Errors in the Intensive Care Unit: A Systematic Review of

Autopsy Studies," *BMJ Quality & Safety* 21, no. 11 (2012): 894–902; Mark L. Graber, "The Incidence of Diagnostic Error in Medicine," *BMJ Quality & Safety* 22 (2013): ii21–ii27; Monica Van Such et al., "Extent of Diagnostic Agreement Among Medical Referrals," *Journal of Evaluation in Clinical Practice* 23, no. 4 (2017): 870–4.

2   https://www.improvediagnosis.org/factors-in-diagnostic-error/.

3   National Academies of Sciences, Engineering, and Medicine, *Improving Diagnosis in Health Care*, National Academies Press, 2016.

4   Mark Olfson et al., "Premature Mortality Among Adults With Schizophrenia in the United States," *JAMA Psychiatry* 72, no. 12 (2015): 1172–81; Shuichi Suetani, Harvey A. Whiteford, and John J. McGrath, "An Urgent Call to Address the Deadly Consequences of Serious Mental Disorders," *JAMA Psychiatry* 72, no. 12 (2015): 1166–7.

5   "Premature Death Among People With Severe Mental Disorders," WHO (accessed December 30, 2018), http://www.who.int/mental_health/management/info_sheet .pdf; Allen Frances, "Having a Severe Mental Illness Means Dying Young," *Huffington Post* (updated February 28, 2015), https://www.huffingtonpost.com/allen-frances /having-a-severe-mental-illness-means-dying-young_b_6369630.html.

6   Joe Burns, "Can Separate Be Equal? Ending the Segregation of Mental Health," *Managed Care* (May 10, 2015), https://www.managedcaremag.com/archives/2015 /5/can-separate-be-equal-ending-segregation-mental-health.

7   Editorial, "Neuroimmune Communication," *Nature Neuroscience* no. 20 (January 2017): 127, https://www.nature.com/articles/nn.4496.

8   Carl Nathan and Aihao Ding, "Nonresolving Inflammation," *Cell* 140, no. 6 (2010): 871–82.

9   Michael L. M. Murphy et al., "Offspring of Parents Who Were Separated and Not Speaking to One Another Have Reduced Resistance to the Common Cold as Adults," *PNAS* 114, no. 25 (2017): 6515–20.

10 Bruce S. McEwen, "Protective and Damaging Effects of Stress Mediators," *New England Journal of Medicine* 38, no. 3 (1998): 171–9; Richard Schulz and Scott R. Beach, "Caregiving as a Risk Factor for Mortality: The Caregiver Health Effects Study," *JAMA* 282, no. 23 (1999): 2215–19; Jos F. Brosschot, William Gerin, and Julian F. Thayer, "The Perseverative Cognition Hypothesis: A Review of Worry, Prolonged Stress-Related Physiological Activation, and Health," *Journal of Psychosomatic Research* 60, no. 2 (2006): 113–24.

11 Phillip T. Marucha, Janice K. Kiecolt-Glaser, and Mehrdad Favagehi, "Mucosal Wound Healing Is Impaired by Examination Stress," *Psychosomatic Medicine* 60, no. 3 (1998): 362–65.

12 Janice K. Kiecolt-Glaser et al., "Hostile Marital Interactions, Proinflammatory Cytokine Production, and Wound Healing," *Archives of General Psychiatry* 62, no. 12 (2005): 1377–84.

13 "Early Experiences Can Alter Gene Expression and Affect Long-Term Development: Working Paper #10." National Scientific Council on the Developing Child, Center on the Developing Child at Harvard University (May 2010), http://developingchild .harvard.edu/wp-content/uploads/2010/05/Early-Experiences-Can-Alter-Gene -Expression-and-Affect-Long-Term-Development.pdf.

14 Jack P. Shonkoff et al., Committee on Psychosocial Aspects of Child and Family Health, and Committee on Early Childhood, Adoption, and Dependent Care, "The Lifelong Effects of Early Childhood Adversity and Toxic Stress," *Pediatrics* 129, no. 1 (2012): e232–e246.

15 Katherine P. Theall et al., "Neighborhood Disorder and Telomeres."

16 Ming-Te Wang and Sarah Kenny, "Longitudinal Links Between Fathers' and Mothers' Harsh Verbal Discipline and Adolescents' Conduct Problems and Depressive Symptoms," *Child Development* 85, no. 3 (2014): 908–23.

17 Rebecca E. Lacey, Meena Kumari, and Anne McMunn, "Parental Separation in Childhood and Adult Inflammation: The Importance of Material and Psychosocial Pathways," *Psychoneuroendocrinology* 38, no. 11 (2013): 2476–84.

18 Lin Yuan et al., "Oxytocin Inhibits Lipopolysaccharide-Induced Inflammation in Microglial Cells and Attenuates Microglial Activation in Lipopolysaccharide-Treated Mice," *Journal of Neuroinflammation* 13, no. 1 (2016): 77.

19 Omar M. E. Abdel-Salam, Ayman R. Baiuomy, and Mahmoud S. Arbid, "Studies on the Anti-Inflammatory Effect of Fluoxetine in the Rat," *Pharmacological Research* 49, no. 2 (2004): 119–31; Joshua Rosenblat and Roger McIntyre, "Bipolar Disorder and Immune Dysfunction: Epidemiological Findings, Proposed Pathophysiology and Clinical Implications," *Brain Sciences* 7, no. 11 (2017): 144; Shunsuke Yamamoto et al., "Haloperidol Suppresses NF-kappaB to Inhibit Lipopolysaccharide-Induced Pro-Inflammatory Response in RAW 264 Cells," *Medical Science Monitor: International Medical Journal of Experimental and Clinical Research* 22 (2016): 367.

20 Fiammetta Cosci, Giovanni A. Fava, and Nicoletta Sonino, "Mood and Anxiety Disorders as Early Manifestations of Medical Illness: A Systematic Review," *Psychotherapy and Psychosomatics* 84, no. 1 (2015): 22–9.

21 National Scientific Council, "Excessive Stress Disrupts the Development of Brain Architecture," *Journal of Children's Services* 9, no. 2 (2014): 143–53; Hillary A. Franke, "Toxic Stress: Effects, Prevention and Treatment," *Children* 1, no. 3 (2014): 390–402.

22 Mazen Sabah, James Mulcahy, and Adam Zeman, "Herpes Simplex Encephalitis," *BMJ* 344 (2012): e3166.

23 Crisanto Diez-Quevedo et al., "Validation and Utility of the Patient Health Questionnaire in Diagnosing Mental Disorders in 1003 General Hospital Spanish Inpatients," *Psychosomatic Medicine* 63, no. 4 (2001): 679–86.

24 Perla Kaliman et al., "Rapid Changes in Histone Deacetylases and Inflammatory Gene Expression in Expert Meditators," *Psychoneuroendocrinology* 40 (2014): 96–107.

25 Marie Kim Wium-Andersen and Sune Fallgaard Nielsen, "Elevated C-Reactive Protein Levels, Psychological Distress, and Depression in 73,131 Individuals," *JAMA Psychiatry* 70, no. 2 (2013): 176–84.

26 Robert H. Schneider et al., "Stress Reduction in the Secondary Prevention of Cardiovascular Disease: Randomized, Controlled Trial of Transcendental Meditation and Health Education in Blacks," *Circulation: Cardiovascular Quality and Outcomes* 5, no. 6 (2012): 750–58.

27 Antoine Lutz et al., "Long-Term Meditators Self-Induce High-Amplitude Gamma Synchrony During Mental Practice," *Proceedings of the National Academy of Sciences* 101, no. 46 (2004): 16369–73.

28 Helen Y. Weng et al., "Compassion Training Alters Altruism and Neural Responses to Suffering," *Psychological Science* 24, no. 7 (2013): 1171–80.

29 Robert A. Emmons and Michael E. McCullough, "Counting Blessings Versus Burdens: An Experimental Investigation of Gratitude and Subjective Well-Being in Daily Life," *Journal of Personality and Social Psychology* 84, no. 2 (2003): 377.

30 Elsie Hui, Bo Tsan-keung Chui, and Jean Woo, "Effects of Dance on Physical and Psychological Well-Being in Older Persons," *Archives of Gerontology and Geriatrics*

49, no. 1 (2009): e45–e50; Agnieszka Z. Burzynska et al., "White Matter Integrity Declined Over 6-Months, but Dance Intervention Improved Integrity of the Fornix of Older Adults," *Frontiers in Aging Neuroscience* 9 (2017): 59.

31 Elissa S. Epel et al., "Accelerated Telomere Shortening in Response to Life Stress," *Proceedings of the National Academy of Sciences* 101, no. 49 (2004): 17312–15.

32 Kelly McGonigal, *The Upside of Stress: Why Stress Is Good for You, and How to Get Good at It* (New York: Penguin, 2016).

33 Hermann Nabi et al., "Increased Risk of Coronary Heart Disease Among Individuals Reporting Adverse Impact of Stress on Their Health: The Whitehall II Prospective Cohort Study," *European Heart Journal* 34, no. 34 (2013): 2697–705.

34 World Health Organization, "Constitution of the World Health Organization, as Adopted by the International Health Conference, New York, 19–22 June 1946; signed on 22 July 1946 by the Representatives of 61 States (Official Records of the World Health Organization, no. 2, p. 100) and Entered into Force on 7 April 1948," *WHO, Geneva, Switzerland* (1948).

35 Martin Prince et al., "No Health Without Mental Health," *The Lancet* 370, no. 9590 (2007): 859–77.

36 Kavitha Kolappa, David C. Henderson, and Sandeep P. Kishore, "No Physical Health Without Mental Health: Lessons Unlearned?," (2013): 3–3a.

CHAPTER TEN

1 "Health for All," National Library of Medicine (last accessed January 6, 2019), https://www.nlm.nih.gov/exhibition/againsttheodds/exhibit/health_for_all.html.

2 "Consensus During the Cold War: Back to Alma-Ata," WHO (last accessed January 6, 2019), https://www.who.int/bulletin/volumes/86/10/08-031008.pdf; Marcos Cueto, "The Origins of Primary Health Care and Selective Primary Health Care," *American Journal of Public Health* 94, no. 11 (2004): 1864–74; Anne-Emanuelle Birn, "Back to Alma-Ata, From 1978 to 2018 and Beyond" (2018): 1153–55.

3 Colby Itkowitz, "The Health 202: Patrick Kennedy Shepherded a Major Mental-Health Bill into Law. Ten Years Later, Big Barriers Remain," *The Washington Post* (October 4, 2018), https://www.washingtonpost.com/news/powerpost/paloma/the-health-202/2018/10/04/the-health-202-patrick-kennedy-shepherded-a-major-mental-hill-bill-into-law-ten-years-later-big-barriers-remain/5bb510121b326b7c8a8d17f5/.

4 "The King Philosophy," The King Center (accessed January 6, 2019), http://www.thekingcenter.org/king-philosophy.

5 World Health Organization, "The Declaration of Alma-Ata. Presented at." In *International Conference on Primary Health Care. Alma-Ata.* (1978).

6 Daqing Zhang and Paul U. Unschuld, "China's Barefoot Doctor: Past, Present, and Future," *The Lancet* 372, no. 9653 (2008): 1865–67.

7 Vikki Valentine, "Health for the Masses: China's "Barefoot Doctors," NPR (November 4, 2005), https://www.npr.org/templates/story/story.php?storyId=4990242; Chunjuan Nancy Wei, "Barefoot Doctors: The Legacy of Chairman Mao's Healthcare," *Wei and Brock* 280 (2013).

8 "The largest U.S. Cities," US Census Bureau, City Mayors Statistics (accessed January 6, 2019), http://www.citymayors.com/gratis/uscities_100.html.

9 "China's Village Doctors Take Great Strides," Bulletin of the World Health Organization, WHO (accessed January 6, 2019), https://www.who.int/bulletin/volumes/86/12/08-021208/en/.

10 To see a documentary about this subject, watch "No Woman No Cry," directed by Christy Turlington Burns (2011).

11 Maternal Health: Advancing the Health of Mothers in the 21st Century, Centers for Disease Control and Prevention (2017), https://www.cdc.gov/chronicdisease/resources/publications/aag/pdf/2016/aag-maternal-health.pdf.

12 Leontine Alkema et al., "Global, Regional, and National Levels and Trends in Maternal Mortality Between 1990 and 2015, With Scenario-Based Projections to 2030: A Systematic Analysis by the UN Maternal Mortality Estimation Inter-Agency Group," *The Lancet* 387, no. 10017 (2016): 462–474; "Maternal Mortality," World Health Organization (February 16, 2018), https://www.who.int/news-room/fact-sheets/detail/maternal-mortality; "The Issue," Every Mother Counts (accessed January 6, 2018), https://everymothercounts.org/our-story/the-issue/ Building US Capacity to Review and Prevent Maternal Deaths (2018). Report from nine maternal mortality review committees. Retrieved from http://reviewtoaction.org/Report_from_Nine_MMRCs.

13 M. A. Bohren et al., "Continuous Support for Women During Childbirth," Cochrane Database of Systematic Reviews (2017), issue 7, Art. No.: CD003766. DOI: 10.1002/14651858.CD003766.pub6, https://www.cochrane.org/CD003766/PREG_continuous-support-women-during-childbirth.

14 Lauren C. Howe and Kari Leibowitz, "Can a Nice Doctor Make Treatments More Effective?," *New York Times* (January 22, 2019), https://www.nytimes.com/2019/01/22/well/live/can-a-nice-doctor-make-treatments-more-effective.html; Kari A. Leibowitz et al., "Physician Assurance Reduces Patient Symptoms in US Adults: An Experimental Study," *Journal of General Internal Medicine* 33, no. 12 (2018): 2051–52.

15 David L. Olds et al., "Long-Term Effects of Home Visitation on Maternal Life Course and Child Abuse and Neglect: Fifteen-Year Follow-Up of a Randomized Trial," *JAMA* 278, no. 8 (1997): 637–43.

16 Ibid., *JAMA* 280, no. 14 (1998): 1238–44.

17 "Mental Illness," Statistics, Mental Health Information, National Institutes of Mental Health (last updated November 2017), https://www.nimh.nih.gov/health/statistics/mental-illness.shtml.

18 Melissa C. Mercado et al., "Trends in Emergency Department Visits for Nonfatal Self-Inflicted Injuries Among Youth Aged 10 to 24 Years in the United States, 2001–2015," *JAMA* 318, no. 19 (2017): 1931–33; Sally C. Curtin, Margaret Warner, and Holly Hedegaard, "Increase in Suicide in the United States, 1999–2014" (2016).

19 "800,000 People Kill Themselves Every Year. What Can We Do?" World Health Organization (October 10, 2018), http://www.who.int/news-room/commentaries/detail/800-000-people-kill-themselves-every-year.-what-can-we-do.

20 Ibid.

21 "Depression," Fact Sheet, World Health Organization (last updated March 22, 2018), http://www.who.int/news-room/fact-sheets/detail/depression.

22 Ibid.

23 Debbie F. Plotnick, "Affording Mental Health Care" (2016): 1144–44.

24 Itkowitz, "The Health 202: Patrick Kennedy."

25 Gary Belkin, executive deputy commissioner at the New York City Department of Health and Mental Hygiene, in discussion with the author (November 2017).

26 "Find a Mental Health First AID course," Mental Health First AID (accessed March 11, 2019), https://www.mentalhealthfirstaid.org/take-a-course/find-a-course/; Born This Way Foundation (accessed March 11, 2019), https://bornthisway.foundation/.

27 Richard Layard, "Look Beyond Number One," *The Guardian* (February 2, 2009), https://www.theguardian.com/commentisfree/2009/feb/03/schools-young-good -childhoods.

28 "2018 Edelman Trust Barometer," Edelman Annual Global Study (January 21, 2018), https://www.edelman.com/trust-barometer/.

29 Wendy Suzuki, "Fear Shrinks Your Brain and Makes You Less Creative," interview by Carolyn Centeno Milton, *Forbes* (April 18, 2018), https://www.forbes.com/sites /carolyncenteno/2018/04/18/fear-shrinks-your-brain-and-makes-you-less-creative /#4b1ab1ef1c6d.

30 Sarah F. Brosnan and Frans BM de Waal, "Monkeys Reject Unequal Pay," *Nature* 425, no. 6955 (2003): 297.

31 Lord Richard Layard, London School of Economics professor emeritus, in discussion with the author (October 2018).

32 _____. "Happiness and Public Policy: A Challenge to the Profession," *The Economic Journal* 116, no. 510 (2006): C24–C33.

33 Myrna M. Weissman et al., "The Changing Rate of Major Depression: Cross-National Comparisons," *JAMA* 268, no. 21 (1992): 3098–105.

34 John Helliwell, Richard Layard, and Jeffrey Sachs, "World Happiness Report" (2012); Richard Layard, "Our Basic Purpose" (filmed September 23, 2014), TEDxOxford, Oxford, England, video, https://www.youtube.com/watch?v=iAZwvTV3CyQ.

35 Richard Layard, *Happiness: Lessons from a New Science* (UK: Penguin, 2011).

36 Richard J. Davidson, "What Does the Prefrontal Cortex 'Do' in Affect: Perspectives on Frontal EEG Asymmetry Research," *Biological Psychology* 67, no. 1–2 (2004): 219–34; Richard J. Davidson et al., "Alterations in Brain and Immune Function Produced by Mindfulness Meditation," *Psychosomatic Medicine* 65, no. 4 (2003): 564–70.

37 "Take the Action for Happiness Pledge," Action for Happiness (accessed January 7, 2019), http://www.actionforhappiness.org/take-action/take-the-action-for -happiness-pledge.

38 Daniel Goleman, "What Really Matters for a Happy and Meaningful Life?" Action for Happiness (July 8, 2015), http://www.actionforhappiness.org/news/what-really -matters-for-a-happy-and-meaningful-life.

39 "Happy Café Network," Action for Happiness (accessed January 22, 2019), http:// www.actionforhappiness.org/happy-cafe.

40 Michelle Dean, "Raise My Consciousness: An Appreciation for the Groovy All-Women Rap Sessions of Yore," *Slate* (March 6, 2013), http://www.slate.com/articles /double_x/doublex/2013/03/sheryl_sandberg_s_idea_of_consciousness_raising_a _lost_art_form.html.

41 Gemma Francis, "Parents Will Have 2,184 Arguments With Their Children Every Year" (July 26, 2018), https://www.swnsdigital.com/2018/07/parents-will-have -2184-arguments-with-their-children-every-year/.

42 Colman McCarthy, journalist and founder of the Center for Teaching Peace, in discussion with the author (November 2018).

43 The King Center, "Philosophy."

44 Borislava Manojlovic, "John Lewis?" Love & Forgiveness in Governance, Seton Hall University School of Diplomacy and International Relations (accessed January 7, 2019), http://blogs.shu.edu/diplomacyresearch/2014/01/20/john-lewis/.

45 Colman McCarthy, "Peaceful Conflict Resolution Teachable," *The Baltimore Sun* (March 15, 1998).

46 Nadia Murad, "Outraged by the Attacks on Yazidis? It Is Time to Help," *New York Times* (February 10, 2018), https://www.nytimes.com/2018/02/10/opinion/sunday/yazidis-islamic-state-rape-genocide.html.

47 Ibid.

48 Nadia Murad and Jenna Krajeski, *The Last Girl: My Story of Captivity, and My Fight Against the Islamic State* (New York: Tim Duggan Books, 2018).

49 "Security Council Requests Creation of Independent Team," United Nations (September 21, 2017), https://www.un.org/press/en/2017/sc12998.doc.htm.

50 "Nadia Murad: 2018 Nobel Peace Prize Laureate," Nadia's Initiative (accessed January 7, 2019), https://nadiasinitiative.org/nadiamurad/.

51 "Who Is Dr. Denis Mukwege?" Dr. Denis Mukwege Foundation (accessed January 7, 2019), https://www.mukwegefoundation.org/about-us/about-dr-denis-mukwege/.

52 Nadia Murad, "I Was an Isis Sex Slave. I Tell My Story Because It Is the Best Weapon I Have," *The Guardian* (October 6, 2018), https://www.theguardian.com/commentisfree/2018/oct/06/nadia-murad-isis-sex-slave-nobel-peace-prize.

53 Colman McCarthy, ed., *Solutions to Violence* (Washington, DC: Center for Teaching Peace, 2001).

CONCLUSION

1 P. K. Hallinan, *Heartprints* (Nashville, TN: Ideals Children's Books, 2015).

2 Kevin Kelly, "Lessons Learned Traveling the World," interview by Tim Ferriss. *Tim Ferriss Show*, June 26, 2018, transcript at https://tim.blog/tag/kevin-kelly/.

AFTERWORD

1 Susan E. Weeks, Eugene E. Harris, and Warren G. Kinzey, "Human Gross Anatomy: A Crucial Time to Encourage Respect and Compassion in Students," *Clinical Anatomy*, no. 1 (1995): 69–79; Herbert M. Swick, "Medical Professionalism and the Clinical Anatomist," *Clinical Anatomy* 19, no. 5 (2006): 393–402.

About the Author

Kelli Harding, MD, MPH, is fascinated by the interplay of the mental, physical, and social dimensions of health. She is an assistant clinical professor of psychiatry at Columbia University Irving Medical Center, where she's trained, studied, worked, and taught for over the past decade and a half. She is a diplomate of the American Board of Psychiatry and Neurology, as well as board certified in the specialty of consultation-liaison psychiatry (mind-body medicine). In addition to teaching and public health roles, Kelli has spent the majority of her career in the emergency room at NewYork-Presbyterian Hospital, Columbia Campus, as an attending physician seeing patients who come in with both medical and behavioral symptoms, including anyone acting odd on the subway or found naked on the street.

Kelli is passionate about improving health for all. She gained a bird's-eye view of American medicine from years of involvement in national health organizations, including the Association of American Medical Colleges, where she served on the national board of directors. In addition to receiving teaching and research awards, she's appeared on the *Today* show, *Good Morning America*, NPR, Oprah.com, Greatest.com, Medscape, WFUV's Cityscape, and in the *New York Times* and *US News & World Report*.

Kelli grew up far outside the city lights near Florida and California beaches, in the Rocky Mountains, and the Nevada desert. Her life changed forever for the better when she sat next to her future husband on a flight to London. They now live in New York City with their three sons Max, Ryan, and Zay, and two guinea pigs, Calypso and Miss Mix-a-Lot.